Fast Facts for the NEW NURSE PRACTITIONER: W Nutshell, 2e (*Aktan*)

Fast Facts for the ER NURSE: Emergency Department Orientation in a Nutshell, 3e (*Buettner*)

Fast Facts About GI AND LIVER DISEASES FOR NURSES: What APRNs Need to Know in a Nutshell (*Chaney*)

Fast Facts for the MEDICAL–SURGICAL NURSE: Clinical Orientation in a Nutshell (*Ciocco*)

Fast Facts on COMBATING NURSE BULLYING, INCIVILITY, AND WORKPLACE VIOLENCE: What Nurses Need to Know in a Nutshell (*Ciocco*)

Fast Facts for the NURSE PRECEPTOR: Keys to Providing a Successful Preceptorship in a Nutshell (*Ciocco*)

Fast Facts for the OPERATING ROOM NURSE: An Orientation and Care Guide in a Nutshell (*Criscitelli*)

Fast Facts for the ANTEPARTUM AND POSTPARTUM NURSE: A Nursing Orientation and Care Guide in a Nutshell (*Davidson*)

Fast Facts for the NEONATAL NURSE: A Nursing Orientation and Care Guide in a Nutshell (*Davidson*)

Fast Facts About PRESSURE ULCER CARE FOR NURSES: How to Prevent, Detect, and Resolve Them in a Nutshell (*Dziedzic*)

Fast Facts for the GERONTOLOGY NURSE: A Nursing Care Guide in a Nutshell (*Eliopoulos*)

Fast Facts for the LONG-TERM CARE NURSE: What Nursing Home and Assisted Living Nurses Need to Know in a Nutshell (*Eliopoulos*)

Fast Facts for the CLINICAL NURSE MANAGER: Managing a Changing Workplace in a Nutshell, 2e (*Fry*)

Fast Facts for EVIDENCE-BASED PRACTICE: Implementing EBP in a Nutshell, 2e (*Godshall*)

Fast Facts for Nurses About HOME INFUSION THERAPY: The Expert's Best Practice Guide in a Nutshell (*Gorski*)

Fast Facts About NURSING AND THE LAW: Law for Nurses in a Nutshell (*Grant, Ballard*)

Fast Facts for the L&D NURSE: Labor & Delivery Orientation in a Nutshell, 2e (*Groll*)

Fast Facts for the RADIOLOGY NURSE: An Orientation and Nursing Care Guide in a Nutshell (*Grossman*)

Fast Facts on ADOLESCENT HEALTH FOR NURSING AND HEALTH PROFESSIONALS: A Care Guide in a Nutshell (*Herrman*)

Fast Facts for the FAITH COMMUNITY NURSE: Implementing FCN/Parish Nursing in a Nutshell (*Hickman*)

Fast Facts for the CARDIAC SURGERY NURSE: Caring for Cardiac Surgery Patients in a Nutshell, 2e (*Hodge*)

Fast Facts About the NURSING PROFESSION: Historical Perspectives in a Nutshell (*Hunt*)

Fast Facts for the CLINICAL NURSING INSTRUCTOR: Clinical Teaching in a Nutshell, 2e (*Kan, Stabler-Haas*)

Fast Facts for the WOUND CARE NURSE: Practical Wound Management in a Nutshell (*Kifer*)

Fast Facts About EKGs FOR NURSES: The Rules of Identifying EKGs in a Nutshell (*Landrum*)

Fast Facts for the CRITICAL CARE NURSE: Critical Care Nursing in a Nutshell (*Landrum*)

Fast Facts for the TRAVEL NURSE: Travel Nursing in a Nutshell (*Landrum*)

Fast Facts for the SCHOOL NURSE: School Nursing in a Nutshell, 2e (*Loschiavo*)

Fast Facts for MANAGING PATIENTS WITH A PSYCHIATRIC DISORDER: What RNs, NPs, and New Psych Nurses Need to Know (*Marshall*)

Fast Facts About CURRICULUM DEVELOPMENT IN NURSING: How to Develop & Evaluate Educational Programs in a Nutshell (*McCoy, Anema*)

Fast Facts for DEMENTIA CARE: What Nurses Need to Know in a Nutshell (*Miller*)

Fast Facts for HEALTH PROMOTION IN NURSING: Promoting Wellness in a Nutshell (*Miller*)

Fast Facts for STROKE CARE NURSING: An Expert Guide in a Nutshell (*Morrison*)

Fast Facts for the MEDICAL OFFICE NURSE: What You Really Need to Know in a Nutshell (*Richmeier*)

Fast Facts for the PEDIATRIC NURSE: An Orientation Guide in a Nutshell (*Rupert, Young*)

Fast Facts About the GYNECOLOGICAL EXAM FOR NURSE PRACTITIONERS: Conducting the GYN Exam in a Nutshell (*Secor, Fantasia*)

Fast Facts for the STUDENT NURSE: Nursing Student Success in a Nutshell (*Stabler-Haas*)

Fast Facts for CAREER SUCCESS IN NURSING: Making the Most of Mentoring in a Nutshell (*Vance*)

Fast Facts for the TRIAGE NURSE: An Orientation and Care Guide in a Nutshell (*Visser, Montejano, Grossman*)

Fast Facts for DEVELOPING A NURSING ACADEMIC PORTFOLIO: What You Really Need to Know in a Nutshell (*Wittmann-Price*)

Fast Facts for the HOSPICE NURSE: A Concise Guide to End-of-Life Care (*Wright*)

Fast Facts for the CLASSROOM NURSING INSTRUCTOR: Classroom Teaching in a Nutshell (*Yoder-Wise, Kowalski*)

Forthcoming FAST FACTS Books

Fast Facts About PTSD: A Guide for Nurses and Other Health Care Professionals (*Adams*)

Fast Facts for the OPERATING ROOM NURSE: An Orientation and Care Guide in a Nutshell, 2e (*Criscitelli*)

Fast Facts for TESTING AND EVALUATION IN NURSING: Teaching Skills in a Nutshell (*Dusaj*)

Fast Facts for the CLINICAL NURSING INSTRUCTOR: Clinical Teaching in a Nutshell, 3e (*Kan, Stabler-Haas*)

Fast Facts for the CRITICAL CARE NURSE: Critical Care Nursing in a Nutshell, 2e (*Landrum*)

Fast Facts About CURRICULUM DEVELOPMENT IN NURSING: How to Develop & Evaluate Educational Programs in a Nutshell, 2e (*McCoy, Anema*)

Fast Facts About the GYNECOLOGIC EXAM: A Professional Guide for NPs, PAs, and Midwives, 2e (*Secor, Fantasia*)

Visit www.springerpub.com to order.

FAST FACTS for
MANAGING PATIENTS WITH A PSYCHIATRIC DISORDER

Brenda Marshall, EdD, APRN, ANEF, is a psychiatric nurse practitioner with a private practice in Oakland, New Jersey, and an associate professor of nursing at William Paterson University, Wayne, New Jersey. She is the author of *Becoming You, An Owner's Manual for Creating Personal Happiness* and has published articles in peer-reviewed journals and as chapters in nursing and psychology textbooks. She has been recognized by multiple national organizations for her innovative teaching approaches in psychiatric nursing. Dr. Marshall is an internationally recognized speaker and a Fulbright Specialist in Mental Health. She has served on multiple national boards and been the president of the American Psychiatric Nurses Association's New Jersey chapter. Her three decades of nursing experience, research, and certifications in psychiatric nursing, administration, addiction management, and psychotherapy have won her the respect of her colleagues in nursing, medicine, and psychology.

FAST FACTS for

MANAGING PATIENTS WITH A PSYCHIATRIC DISORDER

What RNs, NPs, and New Psych Nurses Need to Know

Brenda Marshall, EdD, APRN, ANEF

With special contributions from
Benjamin Evans, DD, DNP, RN, APN
Assistant Professor Graduate Nursing and APN Track Coordinator
Felician University, Lodi, New Jersey

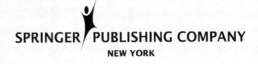

SPRINGER PUBLISHING COMPANY
NEW YORK

Springer Publishing Company, LLC
11 West 42nd Street
New York, NY 10036
www.springerpub.com

Acquisitions Editor: Margaret Zuccarini
Senior Production Editor: Kris Parrish
Compositor: Westchester Publishing Services

ISBN: 978-0-8261-7774-2
ebook ISBN: 978-0-8261-7775-9

17 18 19 20 / 5 4 3 2 1

The author and the publisher of this Work have made every effort to use sources believed to be reliable to provide information that is accurate and compatible with the standards generally accepted at the time of publication. Because medical science is continually advancing, our knowledge base continues to expand. Therefore, as new information becomes available, changes in procedures become necessary. We recommend that the reader always consult current research and specific institutional policies before performing any clinical procedure. The author and publisher shall not be liable for any special, consequential, or exemplary damages resulting, in whole or in part, from the readers' use of, or reliance on, the information contained in this book. The publisher has no responsibility for the persistence or accuracy of URLs for external or third-party Internet websites referred to in this publication and does not guarantee that any content on such websites is, or will remain, accurate or appropriate.

Library of Congress Cataloging-in-Publication Data

Names: Marshall, Brenda, 1951- author. | Evans, Benjamin, 1954- author.
Title: Fast facts for managing patients with a psychiatric disorder : what RNs, NPs, and new psych nurses need to know / Brenda Marshall ; with special contributions from Benjamin Evans.
Description: New York, NY : Springer Publishing Company, LLC, [2018] | Series: Fast facts | Includes bibliographical references.
Identifiers: LCCN 2017026583 (print) | LCCN 2017028068 (ebook) |
    ISBN 9780826177759 (ebook) | ISBN 9780826177742 (hard copy : alk. paper)
Subjects: | MESH: Psychiatric Nursing—methods | Mental Disorders—nursing
Classification: LCC RC440 (ebook) | LCC RC440 (print) | NLM WY 160 |
    DDC 616.89/0231—dc23
LC record available at https://lccn.loc.gov/2017026583

Printed in the United States of America.

Contents

Preface

Patients with psychiatric diagnoses compose some of our most vulnerable global populations, and as the number of people with mental illness continues to grow, the number of specialists and specialized treatment centers is shrinking. One in four adults and one in five children have a mental illness. Regardless of what specialty a nurse chooses in the 21st century, the likelihood of providing care to a person with a psychiatric disorder is inevitable. Nurses, advanced practice and non-advanced practice alike, will be required to:

- Assess and provide care to a person who has mental illness and a concurrent physical disorder or injury
- Work with a child who is experiencing emotional distress with or without a diagnosed psychiatric illness
- Help a patient with chronic pain, perhaps with a psychiatric diagnosis or substance use problem, learn how to live a full life managing pain and staying in recovery
- Support a family who has a loved one who is diagnosed with a mental illness or who may have committed suicide
- Counsel a couple who is expecting a baby and whose family genetic history includes a known mental illness

The specialty of psychiatric nursing follows the general nursing code of ethics and has its own specialty-oriented strategies, interventions, and scope of practice. Many of the more current collaborative research articles demonstrate that having a psychiatric nurse specialist as part of the response team in hospitals, on police forces, and in community planning can promote mental health in the community and decrease negative outcomes for our patients. Although as nurses we use a holistic and collaborative model, when it comes to providing care for the mentally ill, both the patient and the specialty nurse have felt the sting of stigma. As the profession of nursing meets the new demands of the Institute of Medicine's future of nursing suggestions, we will find ourselves creating the policies that focus time, energy, and money on creating a better health care system. Part of that new health care system will be the emerging role of all nurses in dealing with the crisis of mental illness and the emergent opioid epidemic.

This book is divided into five sections:

- *Part I: Mental Health and Mental Illness: What It Is, What It Is Not, and What Nurses Can Do* provides the nurse with general information related to psychiatric diagnosis, prevalence statistics, and theories of etiology. It reviews the basic environmental safety guidelines and discusses ethics in caring for the mentally ill. Finally, it presents the importance of the therapeutic alliance in providing trauma-informed care in a safe environment.

- *Part II: Presentation of Psychiatric Disorders* identifies, and provides brief examination of, seven specific disorder categories that nurses may need for providing safe care to patients on any floor and admitted for any reason, including a psychiatric disorder. These categories include pediatrics and neurodevelopmental disorders, thought disorders (psychosis and the schizophrenia spectrum), mood disorders, anxiety disorders, obsessive compulsive disorder (OCD) and related disorders, trauma and stress, and neurocognitive and neurodegenerative disorders.

- *Part III: Medical Diagnosis and Mental Illness: Symptom Sharing* examines three specific groups of medical diagnoses in which the signs and symptoms of the medical diagnosis share symptoms with a psychiatric diagnosis. Misidentification of these symptoms as purely psychiatric can lead to incorrect treatment of the patient's condition.

- *Part IV: Addictive Disorders* investigates substance use disorders and dual diagnosis (the existence of a substance use disorder with a psychiatric disorder).

- *Part V: Psychiatric/Mental Health Issues: Clinical Setting Challenges* focuses on what the nurse may encounter with patients who have a psychiatric disorder, but who have been admitted to, or are being treated for, a separate medical issue. It closes with suggestions for practice for all nurses in different subspecialties who may be dealing with patients with mental illness.

Every chapter begins with learning objectives. Tables and "Fast Facts in the Spotlight" boxes highlight important factors, adding further information for a fuller understanding of each topic. "Spotlight on the Unit" mini-vignettes present case situations for discussion, focusing on instances in which evidence-based practice meets ethical dilemmas. Each chapter includes references, website resources, and further reading recommendations specific to the chapter topic for those interested in delving deeper.

This *Fast Facts* book is designed for the nonpsychiatric nurse, advanced practice nurse, and the nurse with a psychiatric specialization who want to keep current and share information with others. *Fast Facts About Managing Patients With a Psychiatric Disorder* can serve as an evidence-based, user-friendly resource that will help all nurses provide excellent care to patients with and without a mental illness.

Brenda Marshall

Acknowledgments

There are many thanks to be distributed. I want to thank Dr. Ben Evans for his contribution of Chapters 2 and 3 and for his continuing friendship and collegiality. I want to express my gratitude to Margaret Zuccarini and the editors at Springer, who nursed me through the writing of this book with diligence and patience. Finally, I want to say a heartfelt thank you to my family—Lewis, Olivia, and Megan—who allow me the privacy to write, even on Mother's Day!

I

Mental Health and Mental Illness: What It Is, What It Is Not, and What Nurses Can Do

1

The Continuum of Mental Health

In this chapter, you will learn:

- What is meant by the continuum of mental health
- How theories seek to explain the causes of psychiatric disorders
- What statistics can tell us about psychiatric disorders in the U.S. population
- How mental illness affects life expectancy
- Who is taking care of the psychiatric patients in the community
- Why recovery is so important for patients with psychiatric diagnoses

WHAT IS MEANT BY THE CONTINUUM OF MENTAL HEALTH?

When we talk about a *continuum*, we are referring to the existence of a range of something within a topic. The continuum of mental health spans from mental well-being, where we can think and feel and engage in socially appropriate relationships, to severe mental illness, which denies us the ability to communicate with the world around us. At any given time in our lives, we find ourselves somewhere on this continuum. It can be affected by our physical strength and well-being, environmental conditions, emotional surroundings, ability to find and keep a job, and myriad other topics too numerous to identify. In other words, our mental health changes depending on our ability to cope with our physical and emotional environment.

The World Health Organization (2014) defines mental health as "a state of well-being in which every individual realizes his or her own potential, can cope with the normal stresses of life, can work productively and fruitfully, and is able to make a contribution to her or his community."

THEORIES ON THE DEVELOPMENT OF PSYCHIATRIC DISORDERS

Current theories suggest that our mental health is affected by a variety of factors (see Table 1.1). Research has focused on the following areas:

- Genetics, the DNA that comprises our unique chromosomal identify
- Epigenetics, such as exposure to toxins (smoking, pollution, nutrition) during the 9 months of gestation
- Brain injury and brain abnormalities
- Infectious diseases
- Environmental toxins

Fast Facts in the Spotlight

Anything that causes inflammation in the brain can alter the normal function of the brain. Inflammation may be caused by anomalies of the brain at birth, exposure to toxins, infections, or physical or emotional abuse.

Genetics

Certain psychiatric disorders occur more often in families whose members have a history of these or similar disorders. This finding led researchers to theorize that disorders such as schizophrenia, depression, and bipolar disorder may be linked to multiple specific genetic susceptibilities. When a person with the genetic susceptibility is exposed to stressors such as emotional pressure or biological illness, the gene may be triggered to kindle the psychiatric disease. This

Table 1.1

Brief Overview of Theories	
Genetics	Evolves from genetic composition, thus present at birth
Epigenetics	Evolves from prenatal exposure, thus present at birth
Brain injury and brain abnormalities	Can be genetic, epigenetic, or sustained injury during life; thus present at birth and acquired
Infectious diseases	Can be epigenetic or acquired after birth
Environmental toxins	Can be epigenetic or acquired after birth

could explain why some people in the same family are diagnosed with a mental disorder while others are not.

Epigenetics

Epigenetics is the study of changes caused by external or environmental factors that alter the function of genes. Such changes produce a *marker* or *epigenetic tag.* Epigenetic changes do not alter the actual gene, but rather its function. Epigenetic studies related to mental health have found that drug use by a mother during pregnancy can affect the fetus, child abuse leaves an epigenetic tag, people who commit suicide have an epigenetic tag, and cocaine users have an epigenetic tag that increases the rate of relapse, even when the person has been drug free.

Brain Injury and Brain Abnormalities

Developing a psychiatric disorder after suffering a traumatic brain injury (TBI) is not uncommon. There are famous cases of severe, irreversible personality change after TBI, and more recently cases of depression and suicide in football players who had multiple TBIs have been in the spotlight. In addition to depression and suicide, TBI has been linked to cases of mania, cognitive decline, obsessive compulsive disorder, and psychosis.

Brain abnormalities that interfere with the structure and function of the brain can affect a person's ability to negotiate the emotional landscape. Many neurological conditions that exist due to a brain abnormality include a constellation of psychiatric symptoms. For instance, seizure disorders can be accompanied by attention deficit hyperactive disorder, obsessive compulsive disorder, and tics.

Infectious Disease

It is well documented that syphilis, left untreated, causes brain inflammation and mental illness. Other diseases that can result in mental illness include HIV infection, urinary tract infection, sepsis, herpes, and legionnaire's disease, to name just a few. It was discovered that mothers with herpes simplex type 2 infections during pregnancy were far more likely to have children who developed schizophrenia (Buka, Cannon, Torrey, & Yolken, 2008). Other infections that have been linked to mental illness are streptococcus, parasites, toxoplasmosis, and tapeworm (Brown, Cohen, Harkavy-Friedman, 2001; Ebert & Kotler, 2005).

Environmental Toxins

Lead is an environmental toxin that is known to be related to psychiatric disorders. Children are most often exposed to lead in paint from old buildings. Children with high levels of lead have been found to have a decreased ability to concentrate, and increased impulsivity and antisocial behaviors. Exposure to other environmental toxins increases inflammation in the brain, which in turn causes immune deregulation. This chain of events in the brain is considered to be at the basis of psychiatric disorders triggered by environmental toxins (Galea, Uddin, & Koenen, 2011).

FROM CONCEPTION TO CENTENARIAN

Fast Facts in the Spotlight

Since the days of Aristotle, the famous Greek philosopher, emotional well-being has been connected to engaging in a worthwhile life. Nurses have the ability to help new moms create a safe internal and external environment for their child. We have the capacity to focus the patient on wellness, and support actions that move each patient, from the fetus to the centenarian, toward mental health.

Mental Health of the Parents-to-Be

Pregnancy is a highly stressful time for many parents-to-be. Providing support and information to the parents-to-be can help them start a life that has more than just promise. During pregnancy the mother needs to be able to promote her own psychosocial well-being. This includes learning about best practices for maternal and fetal health, including optimal nutrition, stress reduction, vitamin intake, and reduction of environmental risks. In the United States, all pregnant women are screened for depression and the risk of postpartum depression. Nurses need to know how to help these new mothers get the help they need—before, during, and after gestation.

Children and Mental Illness

One in five children younger than 18 years of age has a diagnosable psychiatric disorder (see Figure 1.1). Socioeconomic status is a risk factor for mental illness: among low-income children aged 12 to 17 years, 21% have a psychiatric disorder. This statistic is even more frightening when one considers that more than half (57%) of the children who are diagnosed with a psychiatric illness come from poor homes. Mental illness occurs disproportionately among children living in poverty, and those from military homes. These children are more likely to end up in the juvenile justice and child welfare systems than children in the general population (Howell, 2004).

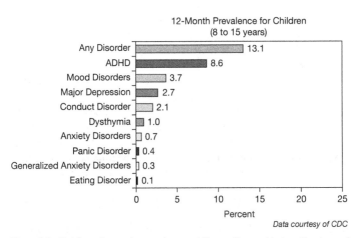

Figure 1.1 Childhood prevalence of mental illness. *Source: National Institute of Mental Health (n.d.-a).*

ADHD, attention deficit hyperactivity disorder.

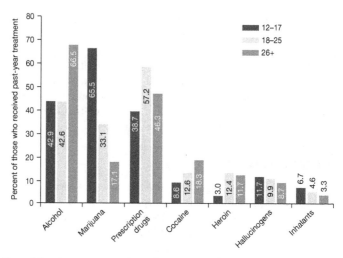

Figure 1.2 Adolescents differ from adults in substances most abused. From National Institute on Drug Abuse (2014); U.S. Department of Health and Human Services (2013).

Adolescents and Young Adults With Mental Illness

Of the youth with mental illness (statistically, one in five children), half will be diagnosed by age 14 and all but a quarter will be diagnosed by age 24. The stigma that is attached to having a mental illness in adolescence and young adulthood often leads those affected to "go underground," hiding their symptoms or using alcohol or illicit drugs to cope, rather than getting the help they need. The National Institute on Drug Abuse identifies early use of substances as a red flag indicator for later drug use/abuse (see Figure 1.2).

Adolescence is a time of experimentation; however, teens who repeatedly use substances have an increased incidence of school failure, HIV infection, psychiatric disorders, and death from overdose (National Institute on Drug Abuse, 2014). The important role played by the school nurse for this population cannot be underestimated.

Prevalence of Mental Illness in U.S. Adults

Eighteen percent of Americans between the ages of 18 and 65 years have a mental illness (see Figure 1.3). This number excludes substance abuse/use disorders. Most of these patients are seen by their primary care provider, in urgent care centers, pharmacy medi-clinics, and

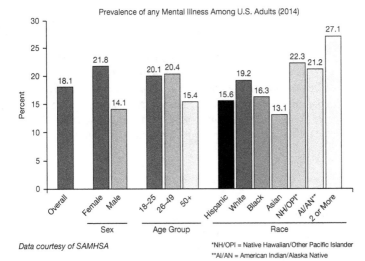

Figure 1.3 Statistics on mental health prevalence in the United States. From National Institute of Mental Health (n.d.-b).

emergency departments. Their first contact will probably be a nurse. The ability to identify the signs and symptoms of the more common psychiatric disorders could be the first step in getting these patients the help they need.

Mental Illness in Seniors

Men older than 65 years of age have a higher rate of suicide than men or women in any other age group. Eighteen percent of seniors have a diagnosable psychiatric disorder, with anxiety being the most common. Often a psychiatric disorder goes untreated, despite effective pharmaceutical and therapeutic interventions. Experiencing frequent mental distress (FMD) is not a normal aging experience and can impact physical health and social engagement. The prevalence of FMD in the 65-and-older population is less than 7%.

Nurses have the opportunity to speak with these patients and listen to their stories and concerns. Although older patients often focus on physical complaints, the nurse who knows the right questions to ask is in the best position to support the wellness of the senior. Brief surveys are available online to aid in this assessment (American Psychiatric Association, 2013).

Fast Facts in the Spotlight

Nurses are in a unique position to be effective facilitators in assisting their patients of any age to get the support and help they need. Patients might think that the anxiety, depression, or phobia they are experiencing is a normal part of their personality, and may never have even thought about getting help. For such patients, a few insightful questions might be the beginning of a better life.

The *International Statistical Classification of Diseases and Related Health Problems*, 10th revision (ICD-10), is a system used worldwide to classify and code diseases and symptoms. Used by both health practitioners and insurance companies, the ICD-10 provides practitioners with descriptions, symptoms, and severity indicators, and provides a foundation for evidence-based, patient population health management. The ICD-10 is referenced throughout the later clinical chapters of this text as an aid to the practitioner.

References

American Psychiatric Association. (2013). Online assessment measures. Retrieved from http://www.psychiatry.org/psychiatrists/practice/dsm/dsm-5/online-assessment-measures

Brown, A. S., Cohen, P., Harkavy-Friedman, J., Babulas, V., Malaspina, D., Gorman, J. M., & Susser, E. S. (2001). Prenatal rubella, premorbid abnormalities, and adult schizophrenia. *Biological Psychiatry, 49*, 473–486.

Buka, S. L., Cannon, T. D., Torrey, E. F., & Yolken, R. H. (2008). Maternal exposure to herpes simplex virus and risk of psychosis among adult offspring. *Biological Psychiatry, 63*(8), 809–815.

Ebert, T., & Kotler, M. (2005). Prenatal exposure to influenza and risk of subsequent development of schizophrenia. *Israeli Medical Association Journal, 7*(1), 35–38.

Galea, S., Uddin, M., & Koenen, K. (2011). The urban environment and mental disorders. *Epigenetics, 6*(4), 400–404. doi:10.4161/epi.6.4.14944

Howell, E. (2004). *Access to children's mental health services under Medicaid and SCHIP.* Washington, DC: Urban Institute.

National Institute on Drug Abuse. (2014). Principles of adolescent substance use disorder treatment: A research-based guide. Retrieved from https://www.drugabuse.gov/publications/principles-adolescent-substance-use-disorder-treatment-research-based-guide/introduction

National Institute of Mental Health. (n.d.-a). Any disorder among children. Retrieved from https://www.nimh.nih.gov/health/statistics/prevalence/any-disorder-among-children.shtml

National Institute of Mental Health. (n.d.-b). Any mental illness (AMI) among U.S. adults. Retrieved from https://www.nimh.nih.gov/health/statistics/prevalence/any-mental-illness-ami-among-us-adults.shtml

U.S. Department of Health and Human Services, Health Resources and Services Administration, Maternal and Child Health Bureau. (2013). *Child health USA 2012*. Rockville, MD: Author.

World Health Organization. (2014). Reprinted from Mental Health: A state of well-being. Retrieved from http://www.who.int/features/factfiles/mental_health/en

2

Environmental Safety and Ethical Care

Benjamin Evans

In this chapter, you will learn:

- How to assess the psychological state of your patient
- What constitutes a safe environment for delivery of psychiatric care
- How the nurse's behavior and attitude can affect the patient's environment
- Which laws guide safe care delivery for the mentally ill patient
- The role of the registered nurse (RN) and advanced practice registered nurse (APRN) in care delivery to patients with psychiatric disorders

ENVIRONMENTAL ISSUES

Assessing the Psychological State of a Patient in the Health Care Environment

Nursing assessment of the health care environment usually occurs on a subconscious level. In everyday life we continually scan our environments for issues that present real or potential threats to our safety. Each environment we enter commands a response from our nervous system. If the environment is dark, noisy, or foul smelling, the environment itself will trigger the reptilian part of our brain—the amygdala, hypothalamus, and brain stem—to respond with an automatic fear/stress response. Experiences accumulated over a lifetime also color our responses, teaching us what is safe and what is threatening.

Nurses are educated, then reinforced through on-the-job training, to identify potential safety issues for the patient and for the staff. When faced with such issues, rather than respond with the "fight, flight, freeze, or submit" response of the reptilian brain, the nurse goes into action to repair and replace, making the environment safe for all.

The patient with a psychiatric disorder, however, presents a different story. The patient may not be able to control the automatic fear response from the sympathetic nervous system. The result is a patient who is on high alert, sensing danger in every corner and from every new provider, with a nervous system preparing for self-defense.

Fast Facts in the Spotlight

There is no such thing as a neutral medical environment. While *we*, as nurses, might be very comfortable in the hospital, emergency department, or medi-clinic, for the patient with a medical or psychiatric problem these are foreign territories. Your ability to evaluate the patient's sense of safety is important. Your response to the patient will become part of the environmental stimuli, establishing it as a safe place or a hostile and dangerous one.

Ensuring a safe environment for nursing assessment and care is always a priority. The following actions help to ensure this need is met:

- *Scan:* Give a quick glance at the environment to establish initial safety.
- *Check:* Assess physical or emotional distress when patient is present.
- *Connect:* Establish the therapeutic alliance, and meet the patient's immediate needs.
- *Secure:* Determine the next steps for provision of safe care in a safe environment.

Initial Scan

If a patient known to have a history of mental illness will be coming onto your unit, it is wise to go into the treatment area (room, cubicle) to be sure things are in order. People diagnosed with a mental illness often have medical problems, sustain injuries, or require urgent and continuous care from health care providers. Prepare your work environment by evaluating the treatment area and determining the availability of all necessities.

When the patient is present, the environmental scan must incorporate a head-to-toe patient assessment, identifying any current physical distress that can help to make the initial contact one that meets the immediate needs of the patient in a professional and empathetic manner.

Areas for Evaluation

■ *Appearance:* Is the patient clean, with good oral hygiene, or unkempt and disheveled?
■ *Initial eye contact:* Does the patient make eye contact with the provider? Is the eye contact constant or does the patient look down or away? Is the patient furtively scanning the room?
■ *Verbal expression:* What is the tone, volume, and cadence of the verbal response? Are the words appropriate? Do they make sense?
■ *Emotional state (affect) as reflected in facial expression:* Is the person emotionally unresponsive to verbal cues (flat affect), or does the facial expression reflect responses, such as anger, fear, or disorientation?
■ *Emotional state (affect) as reflected in body movements:* Is the patient sitting calmly? Or do you notice rigid body movements; nonvoluntary movements (tics); movements suggestive of the patient reacting to a delusion, illusion, or hallucination; or aggressive movements toward staff or others present in the treatment area? Is the patient engaging in anxious pacing? All these movements suggest an elevated level of arousal and should prompt the nurse to take steps to secure the area with additional help.

Evaluating Current Mental Status

In addition to the physical assessment, all patients should be assessed for current mental status. A mental status exam evaluates the patient's appearance, behavior, level of cognitive function, thought processes, and general mental status. Knowing the patient's mental status will help the nurse to prepare the environment so that health care can be provided safely. Several tools are copyrighted and available to clinicians such as the Folstein Mini-Mental Status, the Brief Mental Status Exam, and the Sweet 16 Mental Status exam.

Barriers to Safe Delivery of Care to the Patient With Mental Illness

Biases are a normal part of the human response. Many biases are so much a part of a person's personality, they aren't identified or even considered as biases. A bias can be negative (e.g., when a person, behavior, or disorder is stigmatized), or positive (e.g., when one has a preconceived positive attitude toward people from a particular area). Regardless of whether the bias is negative or positive, it will affect the delivery of care, impacting the nursing philosophy of justice—or equal provision of care to all patients.

SPOTLIGHT ON THE UNIT: BIAS AS A BARRIER TO CARE

Nurse N enters the room of a new patient and is met immediately by a foul odor coming from his direction. Nurse N remembers the night nurse stating that this patient was admitted in the middle of the night after being assaulted. The night nurse noted that the patient is homeless and "probably crazy, too." Without fully entering the room, Nurse N notes that the patient is sleeping. Then, Nurse N steps into the hall and asks the health aide to provide morning care to the patient.

The events outlined in this vignette illustrate how bias, generated in response to the words of another person or to an association of a smell, sound, or visual cue, can interfere with performance of the most fundamental nursing requirements.

- What if the night nurse had stated, "Mr. X was assaulted last night and was admitted to the floor needing q 15 minute checks for LOC?"
- Would Nurse N's response have been different?
- What kind of outcomes could occur though omission of assessment by the nurse?

Stigma: A Negative Attitude Toward Mental Illness

When considering how the nurse responded to the patient in the preceding scenario, keep in mind that stigma is often unconscious.

- What biases relating to homelessness may the nurse have relied on when making an initial judgment about this patient?

- What other factors might have caused this patient to have a foul odor?
  - What if the assault had caused a seizure and resulting loss of bowel control?
  - What if the patient had aspirated from vomiting?

Moving Past Personal Bias

Self-reflection as well as feedback from others should be priorities for the safe provision of nursing care. The feedback from others can serve as a check and balance, as long as the nurse is willing to be honest about the existence of bias as a barrier to care. Diversity training for new employees is one way institutions are seeking to assure equitable care to all patients. Nursing education from diploma to doctoral programs as well as continuing education offerings educate nurses about dealing with special populations and eliminating bias in provision of care.

Safe Environments for the Delivery of Psychiatric Care

All patients deserve health care in safe environments. Caring for any patient will require awareness on the part of the nurse and other health care providers of the actions needed to maintain a safe environment for patients, staff, and visitors.

Psychiatric patients sometimes must deal with more than just the external stimuli of the health care environment. For example, psychotic patients often experience intrusive thoughts, delusions, illusions, or hallucinations that influence their understanding and experience of the environment. In these cases, the patients are also responding to *internal stimuli.*

Health care providers who are called to treat the patient may be unaware that he or she is experiencing these internal stimuli until the initial scan and check is performed. It is important that staff report what the patient is experiencing. These experiences are real to the patient and can be very frightening. They are not something the patient is contriving; they are brain-based symptoms of sensory malfunction.

It is important to understand the differences between these common internal stimuli:

- *Intrusive thought:* A thought that refuses to go away and interferes with the patient's ability to be present (e.g., "I'm going to die, I'm going to die, I'm going to die, I'm going to die").

- *Delusion:* A belief that the patient holds as the truth, despite evidence to the contrary (e.g., the nurse is member of the KGB).
- *Illusion:* An incorrect perception of a real existing item (e.g., the IV tubing is a long worm).
- *Hallucination:* Perceiving or experiencing something as being real that is not present in the environment. This experience can involve any of the senses (e.g., smelling perfume when none exists, seeing a person who has been dead for years, feeling the walls crushing you, tasting peppermint in plain water, or hearing a voice that commands you to jump out of the window).

Patients responding to internal stimuli such as command auditory hallucinations may be fearful and suspicious of staff. Internal voices may be directing them to protect themselves by hitting or hurting the person caring for them. Fearful or anxious patients may need to be placed closer to the care hub or nursing station. Those who are at high risk for running away or leaving the unit (called "elopement" in mental health terms) may need to be placed in a secured or highly visually monitored area.

When managing individuals with psychiatric issues, the nurse must keep safety in focus. Not every patient with a psychiatric diagnosis will be violent; however, if the patient is responding to internal stimuli, the situation can change rapidly. Items that aren't normally considered dangerous can become a weapon. When caring for patients who are known to have violent past experiences, be aware that weapons may be brought in as contraband by the patient or a visitor and hidden from the staff's sight. To ensure the safety of all concerned, the patient's personal belongings, including clothing and bags, should be inspected. The patient should be told what is going to happen, and the staff should inspect the belongings in a "pat-and-shake" manner in front of the patient.

In situations where the patient is highly agitated or very suspicious, nurses might need to work in pairs. Keep in mind that phones, wall-mounted screens and TVs, staplers, pens, and paperclips can all be used as weapons. Good communication with the health care team, ongoing visual monitoring of the patient, and frequent reassuring checks by staff are important to maintain a safe environment.

Nursing Behaviors and Attitudes

Patients with psychiatric disorders are acutely aware of attitudes and often report that they can sense when someone is dismissive or fearful of them. Patients who have manipulative behaviors as part of their symptoms may try to influence staff in an attempt to gain privileges and favors. Patients with paranoia, or highly suspicious thoughts, may take offense to conversations with staff if they feel they are being treated with disrespect.

Maintaining a respectful demeanor, listening to the patient's concerns, and helping the patient to feel safe in the health care environment are very important in establishing a safe therapeutic environment. Misinterpretation of the words and actions of the health care team can escalate an otherwise calm clinical setting. It is for this reason that a number of emergency response teams in Canada and the United States have begun to include psychiatric nurses as part of the response team, to help de-escalate volatile situations.

Nurses in nonpsychiatric settings, such as medical–surgical and emergency departments, are key players in maintaining the safe environment. The nurse who maintains calm, centered balance and speaks in a respectful tone consistently with all patients will be better equipped to identify any shifts in a patient's attitude and behavior in the presence or absence of a psychiatric diagnosis.

Setting Enforceable Limits

Boundaries are established in every health care delivery environment in order to provide safety for patients and staff alike. Nurses are not police. Limits that are established should be shared with the patient and consequences of breaking those limits clearly identified. When a patient is violent, the nurse needs to know the policy for getting help.

The patient will remain for treatment, even if his or her active psychiatric diagnosis is preventing medical intervention at the time. Each health care environment is guided by specific procedures and policies that nurses need to know and follow. No individual provider has the authority to change policy, set limits that are not consistent with the team-based plan of care, or punish a patient whose behaviors are not within the desired norm. The goal of care for all patients is recovery to achieve the patient's highest level of wellness. Patients with any medical problem that threatens life are candidates for experiencing a mental illness. Nursing attitudes and behaviors play a key role in promoting trust, improvement, and a path to recovery.

LEGAL AND ETHICAL ISSUES

Several key issues guide the care of individuals with mental health issues. Historically, the mentally ill suffered mistreatment that prompted the codification of laws and ethical standards to protect all patients. Self-determination, informed consent, the right to be treated in the least restrictive environment, privacy, and the right to refuse treatment are all major components in the care of the individual experiencing mental health/psychiatric disorders.

Self-Determination

The right to self-determination is provided through the Patient Self-Determination Act (PSDA) under the Omnibus Budget Reconciliation Act of 1990. It was enacted on December 1, 1991, and requires that patients be informed on admission that they have the right to be a central part of any health care decisions regarding their care.

Two instruments that help in meeting this requirement are a *durable power of attorney* and a *psychiatric advance directive* (PAD). The PAD allows the individual to identify his or her choices of medications, treatments, and providers. However, the physician can override this declaration at times when the decision-making capacity of the individual is clearly distorted due to his or her mental illness. The override is made through the court.

Other legislation that impacts the care of mentally ill individuals includes the Mental Health Systems Act of 1980, which further protects their rights through the Bill of Rights for Mental Health Patients. Additionally, severely mentally ill individuals have further protections related to employment, housing, public programs, and transportation under the Americans with Disabilities Act (ADA) of 1990.

Informed Consent

The concept of informed consent in mental illness is complicated in the treatment of mental illness. Informed consent ensures that the patient understands both the benefits and costs of treatment. It is problematic when an individual's competence to provide informed consent is compromised by lack of insight or understanding due to the mental disorder. The nurse must know the institution's policies governing informed consent and those with mental illness. Failure to follow such policies can leave the nurse open to litigation.

Right to Be Treated in the Least Restrictive Environment

There are many examples of individuals who were committed to long-term psychiatric treatment for reasons not related to mental health.

Based on these cases, the principle of treatment in the least restrictive environment and manner has been developed (U.S. District Court for the District of Columbia, 1975). This means that individuals cannot be restricted to inpatient treatment if they can be treated successfully on an outpatient basis. Further, patients cannot be forced to take a medication they do not want nor an injectable form of a medication if they are agreeable to an oral medication. Additionally, patients cannot be locked or restrained in a room unless all other lesser restrictive measures have first been tried.

As a quick refresher, there are two paths to admission for the mental health patient—voluntary and involuntary.

1. *Voluntary admission* is likened to any individual who seeks care and admission for a health issue and consents to become an inpatient. All legal rights are retained.
2. *Involuntary admission* or "commitment" procedures are left to the determination of an agency of the state. Procedures vary from state to state or territory. The nurse must be familiar with the procedures for his or her specific state or territory. While procedures vary, there are three common elements to involuntary treatment. One must:
   a. Be mentally disordered
   b. Be a danger to self or others
   c. Be unable to care for one's own basic needs

Right to Refuse Treatment

The incapacity to care for one's own needs includes scenarios in which a patient, due to mental illness, has been deemed incompetent and is unable to accept care that could be lifesaving. Although all patients retain the right to accept or refuse treatment, in an involuntary commitment, periodic court hearings during commitment period deal with these issues—not the nurse. States tend to allow the patient to refuse treatment whether the patient is competent or incompetent. There are usually provisions in state statutes that allow for emergency hospitalizations for further evaluation that range from 48 to 72 hours.

Best Practices

While few lawsuits are filed against mental health care providers, providing appropriate standards of care and documenting such care are key measures to prevent negative outcomes.

Best practices for working with the mentally ill include:

- Using a team approach and including the patient and family (as per patient wishes) in treatment decisions
- Documenting all team and family decisions
- Adhering to agency policy and procedures
- Seeking consultation as needed and recording input
- Evaluating risks when expanding privileges or transferring care
- Utilizing clear, detailed hand-off communication

Fast Facts in the Spotlight

When patients are expressing suicidal or homicidal ideation with a plan, the nurse must provide enhanced security, ongoing visual monitoring, medication as indicated, and variably timed rounding, as well as specific, detailed documentation.

SCOPE OF CARE ISSUES

According to the American Nurses Association's (2007) *Psychiatric-Mental Health Nursing Scope and Standards of Practice*, there are two levels of psychiatric-mental health nursing:

1. Psychiatric-mental health registered nurse (PMH-RN)
2. Psychiatric-mental health advanced practice registered nurse (PMH-APRN)

Table 2.1 outlines the distinctions between the two levels.

The PMH-RN and the PMH-APRN strive to provide safe, effective mental health care with a focus on recovery, wellness, and prevention of further disability. Risk factors, as well as protective factors, must be considered and gauged across the life span. Nurses working with issues of patient mental health, regardless of settings, need to involve other health care providers and gatekeepers as part of a team approach. In this way, the nurse will be able to address the challenging needs and emotional complexities presented in the patient diagnosed with a mental health disorder.

Table 2.1

Levels of Psychiatric Mental Health Nursing

Psychiatric-mental health registered nurse (PMH-RN)	Psychiatric-mental health advanced practice nurse (PMH-APRN)
Nurses from varied educational backgrounds practice in the psychiatric nursing settings with the preferred educational background at the baccalaureate level with credentialing by the American Nurses Credentialing Center (ANCC). These registered nurses demonstrate competence which includes specialized knowledge, skills, and abilities gained through education and experience. This level of practice is characterized by the use of the nursing process to treat individuals with actual or potential mental health problems, promote health and safety, assist in improving coping and maximize strengths while working to prevent further disability.	This level practitioner is a licensed registered nurse who is educated at the master's or doctorate level with specialization in psychiatric-mental health nursing and holds advanced practice specialty certification. The PMH-APRN practice includes the application of competencies, knowledge, and experience to individuals, families, or groups with complex PMH problems and in some states have prescriptive authority. The PMH-APRN works in collaboration with and refers to other health professionals based on client need or PMH-APRN scope of practice. The PMH-APRN is educated to provide psychopharmacology, psychotherapy, case management, program management and development, clinical supervision and consultation. The PMH-APRN may further specialize in areas such as forensic mental health, private individual or group practice, crisis and trauma care, community-based care, and telehealth.

Source: Adapted from American Nurses Association (2007).

Further Reading

Boyd, M. A. (2015). *Psychiatric nursing: Contemporary practice* (5th ed.). Philadelphia, PA: Wolters Kluwer.

Perese, E. F. (2012). *Psychiatric advanced practice nursing: A biopsychosocial foundation for practice.* Philadelphia, PA: F. A. Davis.

Reference

American Nurses Association. (2007). *Psychiatric-mental health nursing: Scope and standards of practice.* Silver Spring, MD: nursesbooks.org.

3

Therapeutic Communication: Establishing a Therapeutic Alliance

Benjamin Evans

In this chapter, you will learn:

- How developing a therapeutic alliance facilitates trust and communication
- How the structured interview guides effective assessment
- How the use of therapeutic communication and active listening elicits concerns
- How trauma-informed care provides a safe therapeutic environment
- How confidentiality rules govern sharing of received information

THERAPEUTIC ALLIANCE

A therapeutic alliance is the felt bond shared between the health care professional (for our purposes, the nurse) and the patient. Through the use of self and professional empathic techniques, the health care provider is able to let the patient know that he or she can be trusted and relied upon and is there to assist the patient during the course of the working relationship. The fact that a patient turns to a nurse does not automatically imply that the patient either trusts or feels valued by the nurse. For example, if the patient senses at any time in the course of the working relationship that the nurse is being dishonest or disingenuous, then all the work in which both have been engaged can be negated and the relationship permanently harmed. Patients tend to "test" the nurse's honesty by asking questions for which they already know the answer, just to see if the nurse is being honest.

The personal attributes of nurses that have been found to contribute positively to the therapeutic alliance include being:

- Flexible
- Respectful
- Confident
- Warm
- Honest
- Open
- Interested

Techniques shown to promote the therapeutic alliance include:

- Reflection
- Accurate interpretation
- Exploration
- Attending to patient experience
- Facilitating the expression of affect (Ackerman & Hilsenroth, 2003)

The nurse who operates from a parental or patriarchal model of superiority usually does not develop a successful therapeutic alliance, possibly impeding the ability to assist the patient in reaching optimal outcomes.

TRAUMA-INFORMED CARE

Many individuals have been subjected to physical, emotional, and spiritual trauma in the course of life. When nurses assist patients who are mentally ill and have a history of trauma, it is important that they take care not to re-traumatize the patient.

Fast Facts in the Spotlight

If a patient with psychosis had past encounters with the police in which he or she was handcuffed and jailed, or taken to an emergency department for commitment to a psychiatric treatment facility, subsequent encounters with police might increase the patient's fear. In such situations, and if faced with seclusion or restraints, the patient can be re-traumatized.

The Substance Abuse and Mental Health Services Administration (2015) provides six key principles of trauma-informed care, as follows:

1. Safety
2. Trustworthiness and transparency
3. Peer support
4. Collaboration and mutuality
5. Empowerment, voice, and choice
6. Cultural, historical, and gender issues

Trauma-informed programs generally identify:

- The survivor's need to be respected, informed, connected, and hopeful regarding his or her own recovery
- The interrelation between trauma and symptoms of trauma, such as substance abuse, eating disorders, depression, and anxiety
- The need to work in a collaborative way with survivors, family, and friends of the survivor, and other human services agencies in a manner that will empower survivors and consumers

It should be noted that key elements in trauma-informed care are safety, trustworthiness, collaboration, empowerment, respect, informed consent, and connectedness. These are the same elements that enhance building the therapeutic alliance. The successful nurse or other health care provider incorporates these elements into care for successful patient outcomes.

CONFIDENTIALITY

Confidentiality in the field of mental health and mental illness is held to a higher standard than in the general medical–surgical and other subspecialty areas. As a result of years of prejudice, inappropriate care strategies, and bias, laws have been enacted to protect patients with mental health issues from having personal health information shared inappropriately. Additionally, based on case law, there are times when the nurse *must* share information to protect others. The nurse must be cognizant of the laws in the state or jurisdiction where practicing. The Health Insurance Portability and Accountability Act (HIPAA) identifies the need for and actions to be taken by the nurse related to a patient's private health information.

In many states, criteria for hospitalization include (a) harm to self, (b) harm to others, or (c) inability to safely care for self (a passive form of the first criterion). Some states also include damage and harm to property or others. In these situations, the nurse may usually share information about the treatment even if the patient refuses consent to do so. As laws vary from state to state, the nurse is advised to know the legal parameters for the state in which he or she is working.

Duty to protect is a concept that emerged from the case of *Tarasoff v. Regents of California* in 1974. The initial hearing set the legal precedent of calling for a "duty to warn" when a patient informs a nurse of intent to harm another. A second hearing in the Supreme Court resulted in a change to "duty to protect" (1976). This requirement called for the nurse to use "reasonable care" to protect an intended victim. Examples of reasonable care include notifying the intended victim, notifying police, or hospitalizing the patient. Many laws in various states have been enacted since this landmark case. Some states allow duty to protect while others prohibit violations of nurse–patient confidentiality under any circumstance. Again, the nurse must know the laws of the state or jurisdiction in which he or she practices.

THE STRUCTURED INTERVIEW

When assessing the patient for mental health–related issues, a structured method helps identify potential problems. A comprehensive mental health assessment is not realistic in most health care environments outside the psychiatric setting; however, all nurses should be able to quickly review the general areas that constitute a mental status check (mini-mental state exam).

Fast Facts in the Spotlight

Quickly assess for mental status by gathering data through patient self-report and clinician observation of the following areas:

- Appearance and behavior
- Motor activity
- Speech
- Mood and affect
- Thought process
- Thought content
- Perceptual disturbances
- Sensorium and cognition

Appearance and Behavior

Do you note any changes from previous encounters? Is the patient groomed and dressed appropriately for the weather, or has hygiene slipped and the appearance become disheveled?

Motor Activity

Is the gait steady? Are there any abnormal gestures, tremors, or tics? Is there evidence of psychomotor retardation (slowing of physical and emotional responses)?

Speech

What are the rate, volume, and coherence? Does the patient speak quickly (possible mania) or slowly (possible depression)? Content of speech is less important than the form.

Mood and Affect

Mood is the patient's internal, self-reported, subjective emotional state whereas affect is the exterior observable state. The nurse might use a simple 1-to-10 scale for more objectivity and ask the patient to rate mood from 1 (sad) to 10 (happy).

Thought Process and Content

What is the rate and flow of thought? Is thought organized and goal directed, or disorganized? Is thought content incoherent; that is, lacking cohesive connections between thoughts? Thought content describes what the patient is thinking. Are delusions or obsessions present? Remember, from Chapter 2, that a delusion is a fixed false belief not in keeping with reality. Is there any suicidal or homicidal ideation? If there is evidence of any thought disorders, the nurse must assess the intensity and specificity for such.

Sensorium and Cognition

Assessing sensorium assesses the patient's level and stability of consciousness. Fluctuation in sensorium may be indicative of delirium. What is the state of the patient's concentration, attention, and memory? These deal with the patient's cognitive status. How is the patient's short- and long-term memory? Remember, questions to assess these areas should take into account the patient's cultural and educational background (see Chapter 2).

A REVIEW OF ACTIVE LISTENING AND THERAPEUTIC COMMUNICATION

Fast Facts in the Spotlight

Barriers to active listening can be:

- Linguistic
- Cultural
- Interpersonal
- Physical
- Organizational

Each of us has at one time or another been in a conversation with someone when they looked at their watch, checked their cellphone messages, or answered a call. In other words, we were not the sole focus of the listener's attention. Dialogue is mutual and balanced listening and response by the individuals involved. To utilize active listening means that the nurse removes distractions, listens to spoken signs and sounds (this is why e-mail communication isn't always ideal), and provides feedback to the speaker that what has been said has been correctly heard and understood. Active listening promotes an increase in mutual understanding, it provides concentration, it constructs meaning, and it responds to and remembers what was said.

Listener qualities that facilitate active listening include respect, acceptance, congruence, concreteness, empathy, and an undivided attention. It should be noted that acceptance does not imply that the nurse accepts all the ideas and material that the speaker sends, especially if the individual is highly mentally disorganized. What it does imply is the acceptance of the speaker as an individual.

In practice, many observers have noted that the nurse can spend quite a bit of time with a patient only to have the patient divulge the real issue just at the end of the session or as the nurse is exiting the patient's area. It may not be feasible to stay longer to address the issue, but the nurse can set a time to return and pick up the issue (unless the patient is addressing harm to self or others, which requires immediate attention).

Fast Facts in the Spotlight

The nurse who is engaged in active listening will be hearing what the patient says and listening to identify the:

- Theme of the conversation
- Supporting ideas
- Physical messages
- Digression from the topic

The following six basic skills should be in every nurse's therapeutic communication toolbox.

Silence

By allowing silence, the listener provides time for the speaker to gather his or her thoughts and pull ideas for the communication together.

Encouragement

Encouragement by the listener sends a message back to the speaker that the listener (nurse) is actively listening and encourages the patient to continue. A simple "go on" or "tell me a little bit more" can offer the patient encouragement.

Clarification

Clarification lets the patient know that the listener has not fully understood what is being communicated, or it allows the listener to hone in on themes that may underlie the communication. A question such as "Can you tell me what you mean by . . . ?" can elicit a clarifying statement.

Paraphrasing

Paraphrasing involves the listener putting into his or her own words what was heard from the patient. This is a way to validate what was heard. If necessary, it can also be used to clarify what was not heard correctly. "So you feel that you are alone and that is the reason for your depression" is a way of paraphrasing a patient's statement that "I feel depressed; life is just gray and holds no future, especially since I am alone."

Reflection

Reflection has two elements: (a) reflection of feelings and (b) reflection of facts. The nurse who is reflecting feelings might state (see previous technique), "You are feeling lonely and depressed," and follow up, "Is that correct?" This is an example of reflection and validation with the patient; the nurse reflects the feeling content and validates that the perception is correct. In reflection of facts, the nurse might state, "You are single and most of your family is deceased, so you feel alone."

Summarization

Summarizing lets the patient know that the nurse "got" the message—its core and all related parts. Summarizing allows for the patient to feel that she or he was really listened to and heard by the nurse. It also allows the nurse to validate that what the patient needed to express was indeed received in the dialogue.

THERAPEUTIC RELATIONSHIPS AND ALLIANCES

Fast Facts in the Spotlight

Every patient deserves to have a therapeutic alliance with the health care provider. This means that health care providers, including nurses, and patients will collaborate with each other in a partnership that focuses on effecting a change that will benefit the patient. In therapy, this change works toward patient recovery, assisting the patient to obtain the best possible outcomes.

There is a myth that therapeutic relationships just happen. They don't. Developing the therapeutic alliance requires strategies and skills that evolve over time, and with practice and guidance. Developing a therapeutic alliance facilitates trust and communication. Therapeutic communication and active listening elicit concerns and assist in assessing need, planning interventions, implementing care, and, it is to be hoped, arriving at quality outcomes.

The nurse ensures that information is gathered in a structured, confidential manner, keeping in mind trauma-informed principles of care, and maintaining patient confidentiality. Developing one's own style of therapeutic communication requires instruction, ongoing guidance, practice, and diligence. The goal of the therapeutic alliance is to be the partner and facilitator of mental, physical, and spiritual health for the patient.

Further Reading

Northrup, G. M. (2005). Tarasoff: Duty to protect (not warn)—Response to a Tale of Two States. *Psychiatry*, *2*(7), 53. Retrieved from http://www.ncbi.nlm.nih.gov/pmc/articles/PMC3000201

Snyderman, D., & Rovner, B. W. (2009). Mental status examination in primary care: A review. *American Family Physician*, *80*(8), 809–814. Retrieved from http://www.aafp.org/afp/2009/1015/p809.html

References

Ackerman, S. J., & Hilsenroth, M. J. (2003). A review of therapist characteristics and techniques positively impacting the therapeutic alliance. *Clinical Psychology Review, 23*, 1–33. doi:10.1016/S0272-7358(02)00146-0

Substance Abuse and Mental Health Services Administration. (2015, August 14). Trauma-informed approach and trauma-specific interventions. Retrieved from http://www.samhsa.gov/nctic/trauma-interventions

II

Presentation of Psychiatric Disorders

4

Pediatrics and Neurodevelopmental Disorders

In this chapter, you will learn:

- Key concepts about the brain, and how brain development is linked to disorders of childhood
- Common neurodevelopmental disorders (NDDs) affecting children and adolescents
- Statistics related to childhood and adolescent mental disorders
- Prevalent specific childhood psychiatric disorders
- Prevalence, etiology, and signs and symptoms of autism spectrum disorder (ASD)

THE BRAIN

One approach to psychiatric disorders is to examine the biological organ of interest, namely, the brain. Not unlike other organs that are the epigenetic center for diseases, the brain is affected by malfunctions during development, causing an impact on mental functioning. Development of the brain, and normal growth over time, may provide clues to different psychiatric disorders. For example, the brain is enlarged in people with autism, normal brain maturation is delayed in those diagnosed with attention deficit hyperactivity disorder (ADHD; National Institute of Mental Health, 2008), and brains of fetuses exposed to the Zika virus fail to thrive in utero.

BRAIN DEVELOPMENT

The brain develops from the third gestational week until a person is in his or her mid-20s. Embryonic tissue (ectoderm) makes up the early nervous system and eventually forms the fetal brain. Development of the brain is dependent on good physical and emotional nourishment in utero and after birth. The brain, like many organs, continues to grow throughout childhood into early adulthood. Anatomical maturation is usually reached in the mid to late 20s. The brain's plasticity, or ability to generate new neurons (neurogenesis), continues over the life span.

NDDs, CHILDHOOD PSYCHIATRIC DISORDERS, AND THE BRAIN

An NDD is caused by an event (genetic or acquired) that interferes with the normal neural growth and development of the brain in utero. There are four identified clinical categories in NDD: (a) developmental delay, (b) attention deficit hyperactive disorder, (c) intellectual disability, and (d) autism spectrum disorders. These categories of NDD are also associated with seizures and schizophrenia, although symptoms of the latter do not appear until adolescence or early adulthood.

The Genetics of NDDs

Two categories of NDDs are differentiated:

1. Rare, genetically based syndromes such as fragile X, Down, Rett, and Angelman syndromes; common symptoms include intellectual disability (ID), seizure disorder, and ASD
2. Idiopathic occurrence of ID, ASD, schizophrenia, and epilepsy

Fast Facts in the Spotlight

NDDs impair many functions that most people take for granted, such as language, mood, and motor control. The burden is felt not only by the individual with NDD, but also by the family and caregivers who will provide support for this person for a lifetime.

STATISTICS

The statistics on pediatric and school-aged psychiatric disorders clearly demonstrate the need for all nurses, regardless of specialty area, to know how to identify, treat, and refer children and their families for diagnostic evaluation and intervention by mental health professionals. As with any medical diagnosis, the earlier a child can be identified with a psychiatric disorder, the better the long-term prognosis will be.

Many people today use the Internet as their diagnostic bible; however, many facts found online are mis-stated. This is true of both self-help websites and provider-oriented sites in the medical and psychiatric fields. As nurses, it is our job to be able to recognize patients in need, identify the problem, assess the facts, and plan an appropriate course of action. Neonatal intensive care unit (NICU) nurses, school nurses, and nurses in medi-clinics and emergency departments all require the same knowledge to identify and refer children and their families to the best evidence-based interventions, whether the problem is physical or psychological in nature.

Mental illness does not discriminate on ethnic or racial grounds, nor does it depend on where a child lives (see Figure 4.1). The Centers for Disease Control and Prevention (CDC) estimates that 13% to 20% of children, or one out of every five, have symptoms of a mental illness each year (Committee on the Prevention of Mental Disorders and Substance Abuse Among Children, Youth, and Young Adults: Research Advances and Promising Interventions, O'Connell, Boat, & Warner, 2009). Almost $250 billion is spent annually on treating psychiatric disorders of childhood.

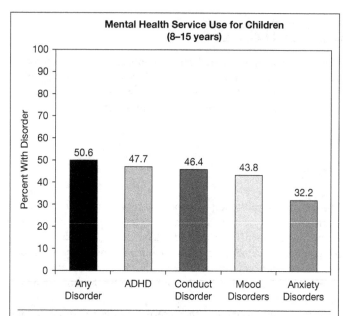

Demographics Associated With Mental Health (MH) Service Use:

- Females are 50% less likely than males to use MH services.
- 12- to 15-year-olds are 90% more likely than 8- to 11-year-olds to use MH services.
- No differences were found between races for mood, anxiety, or conduct disorders. Mexican Americans and other Hispanic youth had significantly lower 12-month rates of ADHD compared to non-Hispanic white youth.

Data courtesy of CDC

Figure 4.1 Mental health service use for children. *Source: National Institute of Mental Health. (n.d.).*

ADHD, attention deficit hyperactivity disorder.

ASD AND DEVELOPMENTAL DISABILITIES

Prevalence

ASD has an estimated prevalence of about 1 in 68 children. It is more common in White children than in Black or Hispanic children, with boys more likely to be diagnosed than girls. ASD is usually diagnosed by age 4 years, with symptoms observable for diagnosis by age 2 (Biao, 2014).

Etiology

ASD is an NDD that commonly manifests early in childhood. According to Gesundheit and Rosenzweig (2016), little is known about the etiology of ASD. It is considered highly heritable, however, and research examining the added impact of environmental factors on genetic expression of this disorder is ongoing (Chaste & Leboyer, 2012).

Signs and Symptoms

- Delay in communication skills; lack of response when name is called
- Responds to questions with unrelated answers
- Delayed or lack of social skills; difficulty understanding feelings (self and others)
- Hyperactivity, impulsivity, reactive behaviors
- May act aggressively, causing injury to self and others
- Resistance to change; obsessive interests
- Difficulty with "pretend games"
- Unusual reactions to stimuli (touch, smell, taste, hearing, vision)
- Unusual patterns of eating and sleeping

SPOTLIGHT ON THE UNIT: INJURED BOY WITH AN NDD IN THE EMERGENCY DEPARTMENT

Mrs. X arrives frantically in the emergency department, her arms filled with a crying 10-month-old and towing an unhappy, bleeding 3-year-old boy behind her. The son hides under the gurney and the baby girl in her arms stops crying. As you interview the mother, she states "Billy is really a brilliant, quirky child. He doesn't mean to hurt his sister, he is just so curious. He was spinning in the living room, like he often does, and he fell on his sister and cut his head on the baby's toy. I'm afraid he broke her arm!" She pulls the blanket back on the baby girl to reveal a small black and blue mark above the elbow. You notice that Billy's cut is still bleeding and call his name, but he does not respond. When his mom reaches for him, he starts yelling and tries to hit her.

- What are the possible problems you are facing?
- What are your thoughts as to the needs of this family?
- What do you do next?

Further Reading

American Psychiatric Association. (2013). *Diagnostic and statistical manual of mental disorders* (5th ed.). Arlington, VA: American Psychiatric Publishing.

Buck, C. (2015, August). *2016 ICD-10: Professional edition*. New York, NY: Saunders.

Cepeda, C. (2010). *Clinical manual for the psychiatric interview of children and adolescents*. Arlington, VA: American Psychiatric Publishing.

Charney, D., & Nestler, E. (Eds.). (2009). *Neurobiology of mental illness*. New York, NY: Oxford University Press.

Halter, M. J., & Varcarolis, E. M. (2014). *Varcarolis' foundations of psychiatric mental health nursing: A clinical approach*. St. Louis, MO: Elsevier.

Johnson, C. P. (2003). Early clinical characteristics of children with autism. In V. B. Gupta (Ed.), *Autistic spectrum disorders in children* (pp. 85–123). New York, NY: Marcel Dekker.

Southam-Gerow, M. (2013). *Emotion regulation in children and adolescents: A practitioner's guide*. New York, NY: Guilford Press.

Weis, R. (2008). *Introduction to abnormal child & adolescent psychology*. Los Angeles, CA: Sage.

Weisz, J. R., & Kazdin, A. E. (Eds.). (2010). *Evidence-based psychotherapies for children and adolescents* (2nd ed.). New York, NY: Guilford Press.

Yearwood, E. L., Pearson, G. S., & Newland, J. A. (2012). *Child and adolescent behavioral health: A resource for advanced practice psychiatric and primary care practitioners in nursing*. West Sussex, United Kingdom: Wiley-Blackwell

References

Biao, J. (2014). Prevalence of autism spectrum disorder among children aged 8 years—Autism and developmental disabilities monitoring network, 11 sites, United States, 2010. *Morbidity and Mortality Weekly Report, 63*(2), 1–14. Retrieved from https://www.cdc.gov/mmwr/pdf/ss/ss6302.pdf

Chaste, P., & Leboyer, M. (2012). Autism risk factors: Genes, environment, and gene-environment interactions. *Dialogues in Clinical Neuroscience, 14*(3), 281–292.

Committee on the Prevention of Mental Disorders and Substance Abuse Among Children, Youth, and Young Adults: Research Advances and Promising Interventions; O'Connell, M. E., Boat, T., & Warner, K. E. (Eds.). (2009). *Preventing mental, emotional, and behavioral disorders among young people: Progress and possibilities*. Washington, DC: National Academies Press. Retrieved from https://www.ncbi.nlm.nih.gov/books/NBK32776

Gesundheit, B., & Rosenzweig, J. P. (2016). Editorial: Autism spectrum disorders (ASD): Searching for the biological basis for behavioral symptoms

and new therapeutic targets. *Frontiers in Neuroscience, 10*, 607. doi:10
.3389/fnins.2016.00607

National Institute of Mental Health. (n.d.). Use of mental health services and treatment among children. Retrieved from http://www.nimh.nih.gov/ health/statistics/prevalence/use-of-mental-health-services-and-treatment -among-children.shtml

National Institute of Mental Health. (2008, May 6). Clues to role of brain development as risk for mental disorders may also lead to better treatments. Retrieved from http:// www.nimh.nih.gov/news/science-news/2008/clues -to-role-of-brain-development-as-risk-for-mental-disorders-may-also-lead -to-better-treatments.shtml

5

Thought Disorders: Psychosis and the Schizophrenia Spectrum

In this chapter, you will learn:

- Statistics related to psychosis and schizophrenia spectrum
- How to recognize the signs and symptoms of psychosis, schizophrenia, and thought disorders
- Prevalent specific thought disorders
- Evaluation of presenting symptoms in patients with thought disorders
- Common medications and therapeutic strategies used to treat thought disorders
- Nursing diagnoses and the *International Classification of Diseases and Related Health Problems*, 10th revision (ICD-10) classifications for thought disorders

STATISTICS

The National Institute of Mental Health (NIMH) statistics on thought disorders (psychosis and schizophrenia spectrum) indicate that about 3% of people living in the United States have a psychotic experience, with 100,000 new (first experience) psychotic events occurring each year in adolescents and young adults (NIMH, 2015). Schizophrenia affects about 1% of U.S. adults (NIMH, n.d.). Schizophrenia spectrum disorders, while not as common, are very disabling and have a significant impact on the individual, family, and community. Although children can be diagnosed with schizophrenia, the average age of onset for symptoms is 16 to 30 years.

Risk factors for schizophrenia identified by the NIMH include:

- Genetic predisposition
- Virus exposure
- Prenatal malnutrition and other in-utero events affecting brain chemistry and structure

Psychosocial factors may be another risk factor. These include but are not limited to perinatal exposure to viruses, inadequate maternal nutrition, and problems during the birthing process (NIMH, 2016).

RECOGNIZING SIGNS AND SYMPTOMS OF SCHIZOPHRENIA SPECTRUM AND OTHER PSYCHOTIC DISORDERS

Thought Disorders

Schizophrenia spectrum disorders present a constellation of symptoms and are characterized by a lack of insight. They are strongly associated with neurocognitive disorders and genetic etiology. The duration of symptoms is important in differentiating among this group of disorders. For example, patients with schizophreniform disorder and schizophrenia may present with the same symptoms; however, in schizophrenia, symptoms have lasted for at least 6 months with 1 month of active symptoms, whereas in schizophreniform disorder, symptoms have lasted 1 to 6 months without significant functional decline (Sadock & Sadock, 2008).

Characteristic Signs

The main characteristic signs of schizophrenia spectrum and psychotic diseases are:

- *Delusions*: Thoughts or beliefs, generally irrational, that are held despite evidence to the contrary
- *Hallucinations*: Experiencing something that is not present, which can affect all senses
- *Disorganized speech*: Jumping from one topic to another without any identifiable connection, sometimes called "word salad," which might include inappropriate repetition of words being said (echolalia)

■ *Disorganized behavior*: Unpredictable behaviors that interfere with normal ability to engage in productive, and even basic self-care

Characteristic Symptoms

These characteristics have been identified in three categories: (a) positive symptoms, (b) negative symptoms, and (c) cognitive symptoms. Each of these categories exists on a continuum from mild to severe and should be evaluated related to the presentation and the chronicity of the disorder.

Positive Symptoms

The positive symptoms are those most commonly associated with schizophrenia spectrum disorders. Patients with positive symptoms present the classic picture of the person who lives outside of reality. They often demonstrate delusional thinking, identify or complain of hallucinations (auditory and visual), have bizarre or unusual thought patterns, and may be engaged in body movements that appear unusual or reflect emotional agitation.

Negative Symptoms

These symptoms are indications of emotional shutdown. The patient may appear expressionless and speak with a flat tone of voice, reflecting a sense of anhedonia (lack of pleasure in life), lack of desire to engage in activities of daily living, and even a lack of desire to talk. These symptoms may be read by family members as depression rather than symptoms of schizophrenia.

Fast Facts in the Spotlight

For a patient to be diagnosed with a thought disorder, specific milestones or social/cognitive deficits must be present and quantified. These include social/occupational dysfunction, specified duration of symptoms, and exclusion of other psychiatric and medical diagnosis that could have the same presentation. Unless you are a nurse practitioner, you should not be providing a medical/psychiatric diagnosis for the patient. Your relationship with and keen observation of your patient, however, will be invaluable.

Cognitive Symptoms

These symptoms indicate the patient's reduced ability to access specific executive brain functioning. The patient experiencing these symptoms may have difficulty remembering things, understanding commands or information, or making decisions.

Evaluating Presenting Symptoms

When a patient presents with signs and symptoms of a thought disorder, it is important to look at certain aspects of the presentation. For example, tempo or acute onset of symptoms can help distinguish schizophrenia spectrum disorder from acute head trauma, delirium, a drug side effect, an infection, or a neurological disorder. Another important aspect in correctly identifying whether the disordered thought and behavioral presentation are characteristic of psychosis is to look at the prior history of the patient, the existence of other psychiatric disorders that might have psychotic features, or any other preexisting brain disorders (e.g., Alzheimer's disease or multiple sclerosis).

Think about the individual in front of you: his or her age, sex, education, socioeconomic and educational status, and cultural norms. If possible, elicit a family history of mental illness, vascular disorders, infections and inflammatory diseases, recent travel, nutrition, and sleep patterns.

Many patients will not be comfortable sharing information about drug or alcohol use if they believe they will be judged or punished for use. It is imperative that the patient understand the need for honesty and feel safe and comfortable sharing his or her substance use history. Withdrawal from medications (legal and illegal), as well as use of certain drugs, can mimic a psychotic event. In all situations, maintaining a safe environment, open airway, and access to emergency interventions can be lifesaving.

Schizophrenic patients present the nurse with specific needs for care. Multiple nursing diagnoses, which specifically reflect the unique and specific needs of the patient, can address symptoms of each of the types of thought disorders.

PREVALENT SPECIFIC THOUGHT DISORDERS

Schizophreniform disorders are categorized for purposes of diagnosis as mild, moderate, or severe, depending on a number of factors including intensity of presenting symptoms. The characteristics and deficits previously identified are evaluated for severity, and it is noted how many of these symptoms are presented by the patient. ICD-10 guidelines for differentiating these disorders follow.

ICD-10 Definitions

- *Schizophrenia*—A spectrum of mental disorders where a person's ability to perceive reality is affected. This disorder affects the capacity to understand and provide social/emotional responses that would be considered acceptable. People experiencing symptoms of schizophrenia might have auditory, tactile, visual, olfactory, and taste disturbances; hearing, seeing feeling, smelling, and tasting things that are not real. The person's ability for social/emotional communication can also be affected, presenting as an inability to respond with proper, intelligible speech patterns (disorganized speech) or with appropriate emotional or social behaviors. These symptoms often can lead to the person's withdrawal from society. The disorder is chronic, and severe, usually starting in the late teens or early 20s with unusual thoughts and perceptions as well as hallucinations. The duration of this disorder is at least 6 months.

- *Schizoaffective disorder*—This disorder includes two sets of symptoms. The person will have the symptoms of a mood disorder, like bipolar disorder, and also of schizophrenia during the active portion of the disorder. When the patient is not experiencing the symptoms of the mood disorder, the symptoms of the psychosis, inclusive of hallucinations and delusions persist.

- *Schizophreniform disorder*—This disorder has a different duration from the diagnosis of schizophrenia, in that the diagnosis includes a duration between 1 and 6 months. This disorder is less debilitating in its impact on functioning in daily living, including job and social/emotional arenas.

- *Delusional disorder*—Delusions are untrue beliefs that are held despite evidence to the contrary. A person with a delusional disorder must hold the delusion for over a month, and not be diagnosed with schizophrenia or a mood disorder. The delusion that is held is not one that substantially interferes with the person's ability to carry on activities of daily living.

This disorder is chronic and can be identified in both psychotic and nonpsychotic patients, with presenting symptoms of delusions of jealousy, persecution and paranoia.

- *Brief psychotic disorder*—This disorder presents as schizophrenia, with the symptoms of hallucinations, delusions, and impairment in thoughts and communication, but it resolves in less than one month.
- *Catatonia*—This disorder causes a disturbance in mobility, reflected in the person's loss of control over physical movement or posture. This may be represented by loss of (or excessive) motor activity, an inability to speak (mutism), an engagement in intense negative attitudes or speech, and the mirroring of words (echolalia) or movements (echopraxia).

COMMON MEDICATIONS USED TO TREAT PSYCHOTIC DISORDERS

Antipsychotic medications are central to the treatment of patients with psychotic disorders. Any one of a number of first- and second-generation agents may be prescribed, depending on the severity of the patient's symptoms.

First-Generation Antipsychotics (Neuroleptics)

All antipsychotic drugs are associated with significant side effects. First-generation antipsychotics have a high likelihood of causing cognitive slowing or impairment, and movement disorders that include extrapyramidal side effects and tardive dyskinesia. Commonly used drugs in this class are:

- Haloperidol (Haldol)
- Loxapine (Loxitane)
- Chlorpromazine (Thorazine)
- Thioridazine (Mellaril)

Second-Generation Antipsychotics

Second-generation antipsychotics, too, have a high likelihood of causing cognitive slowing or impairment and metabolic syndrome. Commonly used drugs in this class are:

- Aripiprazole (Abilify)
- Clozapine (Clozaril)
- Ziprasidone (Geodon)
- Risperidone (Risperdal)
- Quetiapine (Seroquel)
- Olanzapine (Zyprexa)

THERAPEUTIC AND ENVIRONMENTAL STRATEGIES USED TO TREAT THOUGHT DISORDERS

Psychosocial Interventions

- *Cognitive behavioral therapy (CBT)* works by using thoughts and behaviors on emotions. It is a solution-focused therapy that increases the patient's ability to cope.
- *Cognitive remediation therapy* can be helpful in improving attention, working memory, and executive functioning.
- *Psychoeducation* increases illness awareness, self-management skills, habit regularity, and recognition of early warning signs of relapse (Colom, 2014).
- *Psychodynamic therapy* examines past problems and unresolved struggles and the impact those experiences are having on the person's present experience.

Client-Centered, Supportive, and Insight-Oriented Psychotherapy

- *Behavior modification:* Desired behaviors are reinforced using a reward system (e.g., token economy).
- *Family intervention:* The family meets together to identify needs, acquire skills to deal with the disorder, provide support to family members, and provide ongoing psychoeducation.

MATCHING NURSING DIAGNOSIS AND MEDICAL DIAGNOSIS

Table 5.1 correlates nursing diagnoses with the ICD-10 codes for thought disorders.

Table 5.1

Nursing Diagnoses and ICD-10 Nomenclature for Thought Disorders	
Nursing diagnoses	ICD-10 codes
Altered thought process	Schizotypal personality disorder (F21)
Social isolation	Delusional disorder (F22)
Sensory and perceptual alterations related to hallucinations	Brief psychotic disorder (F23)
	Schizophreniform disorder (F20.81)
Impaired verbal communication	Schizoaffective disorder, bipolar type (F25.0)
Ineffective individual coping	Schizoaffective disorder, depressive type (F25.1)
Risk for violence	
	Schizophrenia (F20.9)

Sources: Herdman & NANDA (2012); ICD10Data.com (n.d.).

SPOTLIGHT ON THE UNIT: ADOLESCENT BOY ON ORTHOPEDIC FLOOR AFTER A BIKING INJURY

A patient on your floor, Patrick, is calling for the nurse; his leg has just been casted after a fracture to his tibia. His mother comes to the nursing station stating that her son is talking "in tongues" and she believes that he must have been given some drug for his pain that has made him act "crazy." You check the chart and see that he has not requested any medications, nor has he been given any. You go to the room and find his father there, watching TV. Patrick, speaking in a loud voice and staring at the upper corner of the room, says "It doesn't matter what you think, XANDIDO, I will not follow your command!" He looks frightened. His father continues to watch TV. You ask, "Patrick, who are you talking to?" His father responds, "Ignore him. He does this to upset us. Like there are other people in the room . . . he's been worse lately, though."

- What are the possible problems you are facing?
- What is the differential diagnosis?
- What kinds of evaluations do you think Patrick needs?
- Whom do you think you should call for a referral and evaluation?
- What possible safety issues might you have to consider?

Further Reading

American Psychiatric Association. (2013). *Diagnostic and statistical manual of mental disorders* (5th ed.). Arlington, VA: American Psychiatric Publishing.

Buck, C. (2015, August). *2016 ICD-10: Professional edition.* New York, NY: Saunders.

Chien, W. T., Leung, S. F., Yeung, F. K., & Wong, W. K. (2013). Current approaches to treatments for schizophrenia spectrum disorders, part II: Psychosocial interventions and patient-focused perspectives in psychiatric care. *Neuropsychiatric Disease and Treatment, 9*, 1463–1481. doi:10.2147/NDT.S49263

Halter, M. J., & Varcarolis, E. M. (2014). *Varcarolis' foundations of psychiatric mental health nursing: A clinical approach.* St. Louis, MO: Elsevier.

References

Colom, F. (2014). The evolution of psychoeducation for bipolar disorder: From lithium clinics to integrative psychoeducation. *World Psychiatry, 13*(1), 90–92. doi:10.1002/wps.20091

Herdman, T. H., & North American Nursing Diagnosis Association. (2012). *Nursing diagnoses: Definitions & classification 2012–2014.* Chichester, United Kingdom: Wiley-Blackwell.

ICD10Data.com. (n.d.). Retrieved from http://www.icd10data.com

National Institute of Mental Health. (n.d.). Schizophrenia. Retrieved from https://www.nimh.nih.gov/health/statistics/prevalence/schizophrenia.shtml

National Institute of Mental Health. (2015). Fact sheet: First episode psychosis. Retrieved from https://www.nimh.nih.gov/health/topics/schizophrenia/raise/fact-sheet-first-episode-psychosis.shtml

National Institute of Mental Health. (2016). Schizophrenia. Retrieved from https://www.nimh.nih.gov/health/publications/schizophrenia-booklet/nih-15-3517_151858.pdf

Sadock, B. J., & Saddock, V. A. (2008). *Kaplan & Sadock's Concise textbook of clinical psychiatry* (3rd ed.). Philadelphia, PA: Lippincott Williams & Wilkins.

6

Mood Disorders

In this chapter, you will learn:

- Statistics related to mood disorders, including major depressive disorder (MDD), bipolar disorder (BPD), and other related mood disorders
- How to recognize the signs and symptoms of MDD, BPD, and related mood disorders
- Prevalent specific depressive, bipolar, and related disorders
- Evaluation of presenting symptoms in patients with MDD and BPD
- Common medications and therapeutic strategies used to treat MDD and BPD
- Nursing diagnoses and the *International Classification of Diseases and Related Health Problems*, 10th revision (ICD-10) classifications for depressive, bipolar, and related mood disorders

STATISTICS

Mood disorders are those mental illnesses that affect a person's emotional makeup. The diagnostic category in the ICD-10 spans from F30 through F39 and includes MDD, manic episode, BPD, persistent mood disorders, and unspecified mood disorder. Each of the disorders is diagnosed by level of severity, ranging from mild to severe, which is indicated by the numbers that follow the decimal point in the diagnostic code.

The yearly prevalence in American adults of any kind of mood disorder is 9.5%, and the lifetime prevalence is almost 21%, with the average age of onset at 30 years. Almost half the cases of mood disorder are considered to be severe (see Figure 6.1). Half of all Americans diagnosed with a mood disorder receive treatment.

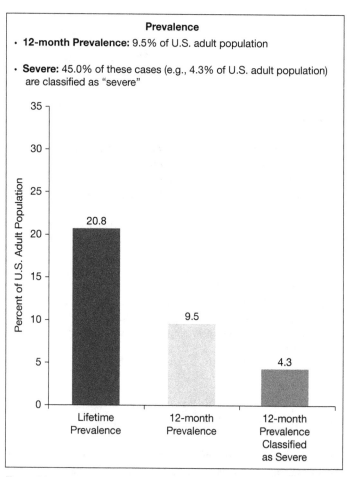

Figure 6.1 Prevalence of any mood disorder among American adults. *Source: National Institute of Mental Health (n.d.).*

DEPRESSIVE DISORDERS

According to the Centers for Disease Control and Prevention (CDC), depression affects approximately 7.6% of Americans over the age of 12 (see Figure 6.2). It has been identified as the major cause of disability for Americans between the ages of 15 and 44 years, and is the most common of all mental disorders. Depression affects women in greater numbers than men, with a mean age of onset of 32 years (American Psychological Association, 2017). Depression is more than twice as likely to affect those below or just at the poverty level, with depressive symptoms identified as serious for almost 43% of those affected. About one-third of individuals with severe depression seek and receive mental health interventions (Pratt & Brody, 2014).

OVERVIEW OF DEPRESSIVE DISORDERS

Major depressive disorder (MDD) is differentiated into MDD single episode, which also includes premenstrual dysphoric disorder, and MDD recurrent. Within each category there are multiple specifiers to distinguish the type of depression as determined by the accompanying symptoms.

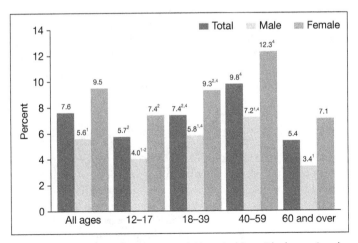

Figure 6.2 Percentage of persons aged 12 and older with depression, by age and sex: United States, 2009–2012. *Source: Pratt and Brody (2014).*

Cardinal Symptoms of Depression

Some of the cardinal symptoms of depression include the following, lasting persistently over a 2-week period:

- Fatigue or complaints of lack of energy
- Sadness, empty feelings, or anxiety
- Disrupted sleep (difficulty falling asleep, staying asleep, or excessive sleeping)
- Loss of interest in activities previously enjoyed
- Change in appetite (loss of appetite or excessive eating) causing weight loss or gain
- A sense of worthlessness or guilt
- Somatic complaints (stomach aches, headaches, muscle pains) without physical evidence of a cause
- Cognitive changes (slow to remember; difficulty making decisions or concentrating)
- Thoughts of suicide, death, or self-harm

Risk Factors for Depression

There is a genetic component to depression; first-degree relatives of a person with MDD are twice as likely to develop the disorder. Temperament and environment are also factors in the development of depression. Individuals with neurotic tendencies (i.e., easily complaining about life, usually negative about the future) and those with lower levels of resilience to life stressors are at higher risk for developing depression. Environmental factors, including but not limited to maltreatment in childhood, trauma, chronic medical conditions, and persistent stress, can also be risk factors for later development of depression.

Suicide

Suicide is the most serious of all risks associated with depression, and the potential for a suicide attempt must always be considered. Suicide among American adults occurs at a rate of 12.6 per 100,000, meaning that one person commits suicide about every 13 minutes (CDC, 2013). It is always important to ask a person who appears to be hopeless, and who talks about self-harm or suicide, the following questions:

- Do you want to harm or kill yourself? (Do they have the idea?)
- Do you know how you might do it? (Do they have a plan?)

- Are you able to get what you need to do it? (Do they have the means?)

Threat of suicide should never be ignored. Sixty-four percent of people who try to kill themselves visited a doctor in the month before the attempt, and almost 40% have seen their health care provider the week before (Ahmedani, 2015).

RECOGNIZING SIGNS AND SYMPTOMS OF DEPRESSIVE DISORDERS

ICD-10 Definitions

The ICD-10 guidelines for differentiating depressive disorders follow.

- There are over 20 million people in America diagnosed with depression. Many people do not realize how serious a diagnosis depression is, or that the person cannot "snap out" of it because they do not have control over it. Like any other medical diagnosis, left untreated, it will not self-resolve and can have a negative impact on activities of daily living (2016 ICD-10 Diagnosis Code F 32.9)
  - Major depressive disorder (single episode) is diagnosed based on level of severity (mild to moderate, F32.0–32.1; severe without or with the presence of psychotic features, F32.2, F32.3) and whether the symptoms are in partial or full remission (F32.4, F32.5). Premenstrual dysphoric disorder and other specified or unspecified depressions are also included in this category (F32.81. F32.89, F32.9).
  - Major depression recurrent is a separate diagnosis (F33.0– 33.9) but shares the same presentation as single episode and the diagnostic indicators from mild to severe with psychotic features. Recurrent depression, also known as "monopolar depression," is diagnosed when a person has had at least one other depressive episode lasting a minimum of 2 weeks, then after a period of 2 months experiences another episode, without having any mood elevation (hypomania or mania) between depressive events (American Academy of Professional Coders, n.d.).

Table 6.1

Symptoms of Depressive Disorders	
Major depressive disorder (32.0–33.9)	**Persistent depressive disorder: Dysthymia (F34.1)**
Symptoms the nurse might see: ■ Tearfulness ■ Lack of energy ■ Weight gain or loss ■ Psychomotor retardation ■ May or may not have psychotic features, depending on severity	*Symptoms the nurse might see:* ■ Many of the same symptoms as major depressive disorder (MDD) but milder ■ Will not have psychotic features
Symptoms the patient will express: ■ Being sad, tired, unable to enjoy normally enjoyable things ■ Somatic complaints with no physical cause	*Symptoms the patient will express:* ■ Same as the person with MMD ■ Having these feelings for the majority of each day for at least 2 years in adults and for 1 year in children or adolescents

■ *Persistent mood disorder (dysthymia)—ICD-10 code F34.1 definition:* "A term used for any state of depression that is not psychotic. An affective disorder manifested by either a dysphoric mood or loss of interest or pleasure in usual activities. The mood disturbance is prominent and relatively persistent" ("2017 ICD-10-CM Diagnosis Code F34.1").

A thorough history is necessary to differentiate the symptoms of MDD and persistent mood disorder (dysthymia). Refer to Table 6.1.

MEDICATIONS USED TO TREAT DEPRESSIVE DISORDERS

Medications are used to treat depression, but some medications can actually precipitate depressive symptoms. Many drugs used for recreational purposes (e.g., alcohol, marijuana, cocaine, and opiates) as well as some of those for hypertension (e.g., propranolol) and gastrointestinal disorders (e.g., cimetidine) can cause symptoms of depression. It is important to obtain a careful medical history from all patients, especially those who present with symptoms of depression, to rule out an underlying cause for the symptoms that is unrelated to mental illness. The list below includes some of the common medications used to treat depression. It is important to remember that each pharmacological antidepressant treatment must be examined individually for effects, dosing, and side effects.

- *Selective serotonin reuptake inhibitors (SSRIs):* Sertraline (Zoloft), fluoxetine (Prozac), escitalopram (Lexapro), citalopram (Celexa), paroxetine (Paxil), fluvoxamine (Luvox)
- *Serotonin and norepinephrine reuptake inhibitors (SNRIs):* Desvenlafaxine (Pristiq), duloxetine (Cymbalta), venlafaxine (Effexor XR)
- *Tricyclic antidepressants (TCAs):* Clomipramine (Anafranil), imipramine (Tofranil), nortriptyline (Pamelor)
- *Tetracyclic antidepressants:* Maprotiline
- *Dopamine reuptake blockers:* Bupropion (Wellbutrin)
- *Monoamine oxidase inhibitors (MAOIs):* Isocarboxazid (Marplan), phenelzine (Nardil), tranylcypromine (Parnate), selegiline (Emsam)
- *5-HT$_{1A}$ receptor antagonist:* Vilazodone (Viibryd)
- *5-HT$_2$ receptor antagonists:* Nefazodone, trazodone (Oleptro)
- *5-HT$_3$ receptor antagonist:* Vortioxetine (Brintellix)
- *Noradrenergic antagonists:* Mirtazapine (Remeron)
- *Prescription-strength vitamins:* L-Methylfolate (Enlyte, Enbrace)
- *Over-the-counter (OTC) medications:* St John's wort, Sam-e

THERAPEUTIC AND ENVIRONMENTAL STRATEGIES USED TO TREAT DEPRESSIVE DISORDERS

Multiple diverse psychotherapeutic and environmental strategies are available to help the person with a depressive disorder. Psychotherapy focuses on facilitating the acquisition of skills and insight that assist the patient in changing the behaviors, emotions, and thoughts that underlie the symptoms of depression. It can be delivered to the individual, the family, or in a group setting; some forms of psychotherapy are provided in person, but many can be accessed online or by telephone. The person who provides psychotherapy is usually a licensed, trained therapist. Knowing the different kinds of therapies and the therapists who practice them is important when referring patients.

Psychotherapy

- *Cognitive behavioral therapy (CBT)* works by using thoughts and behaviors on emotions. It is a solution-focused therapy that increases the patient's ability to cope.
- *Interpersonal psychotherapy (IPT)* is a brief intervention that specifically focuses on the interpersonal issues and problems experienced by the person with depression.
- *Psychodynamic therapy* examines past problems and unresolved struggles and the impact those experiences are having on the person's present experience.

Hospital-Based Treatments

Brain stimulation may be provided using the following techniques:

- *Vagus nerve stimulation (VNS)* involves electrical stimulation of the vagus nerve from an implanted device located in the chest under the skin.
- *Electroconvulsive therapy (ECT)* is designed to induce a seizure. It is used in severe, treatment-resistant depression and is sometimes indicated in pregnancy. ECT is done in a clinic or hospital where the patient can be given anesthesia prior to the seizure, and monitored posttreatment.

Environmental Ecotherapies and Strategies

Naturalistic methods have been demonstrated to be effective in reducing the symptoms of depression. These approaches include relaxation techniques, mindfulness, meditation, yoga, and tai chi. Researchers have studied the effect of yoga on anxiety and depression and suggested that these practices are successful in modulating the stress response that can fuel depression. After 3 months of practicing yoga, participants in one study experienced a 50% reduction in their symptoms of depression (Harvard Health Publications, 2009).

MATCHING NURSING DIAGNOSIS AND MEDICAL DIAGNOSIS

Table 6.2 correlates nursing diagnoses with the ICD-10 codes for depressive disorders.

Table 6.2

Nursing Diagnoses and ICD-10 Nomenclature for Depressive Disorders

Nursing diagnoses	ICD-10 codes
Risk for suicide	MDD single episode (F32)
Complicated grieving	MDD recurrent (F33)
Social isolation/impaired social interaction	Dysthymia: Persistent mood (affective) disorders (F34.1)
Powerlessness	
Low self-esteem	
Self-care deficits	
Disturbed sleep pattern	
Imbalanced nutrition	

Sources: Herdman & NANDA (2012); ICD10Data.com (n.d.).

SPOTLIGHT ON THE UNIT: YOUNG WOMAN IN THE LOCAL MEDI-CENTER

Jaxin, a 19-year-old engineering student, drags herself into the local medi-center, again. She comes in with different somatic complaints on a regular basis, sitting and talking to the nurse on duty. Previously an "A" student and active on the improvisational acting team, Jaxin is now on academic probation due to missed assignments and multiple class absences. She explains that she has dropped out of all club activities and has lost 15 pounds in the last month. Her multiple complaints, from abdominal pain to recurrent headaches, have all been evaluated, but all of her tests have come back normal. She has difficulty maintaining eye contact, and when she does, she becomes tearful and unable to talk. Jaxin explains that she has been very sad lately, thinking about how hard it will be to get a job and live on her own. She says, "I'm just not as smart as my classmates, and they are even having a hard time getting research positions. I'll never get a job, and my parents will be so disappointed with me, I'm such a burden . . . they would be better off

(continued)

without me. Between my school loans and even just needing money for food, I'm a great burden to everyone. I wish I was never born."

- What are the possible problems you are facing?
- What is the differential diagnosis?
- What are the nursing diagnoses?
- To whom should Jaxin be referred?
- What is the most pressing problem that Jaxin may be facing at present?
- What specific questions do you need to ask to determine if Jaxin is safe to leave your office?
- What do you do next?

BIPOLAR AND RELATED DISORDERS

The National Institute of Mental Health (NIMH) reports the adult prevalence of bipolar disorder (BPD) at more than 2.5% (nearly 6 million adults), with more than 82% of cases classified as severe (see Figure 6.3). The average age of onset is 25 years. Unfortunately, only slightly more than half of patients receive even minimally adequate treatment (Kessler et al., 2005).

OVERVIEW OF BPD

Bipolar spectrum symptoms range from the extreme high of mania, in which the person is very excited, energetic, risk taking, impulsive, and elated, to the intense depth of depression, in which any energy expenditure is too much. These experiences are known as "mood episodes" and are far more extreme than the typical mood changes normally experienced by average individuals. It is believed that three neurotransmitters—serotonin, noradrenaline, and dopamine—are involved in BPD. Studies have shown a genetic link in BPD, and family members of a person with BPD are more likely to develop the disease. Environmental factors also influence its development. Children of alcoholics and substance abusers, and those with frequent mood swings and impulsive behavior, are at higher risk of developing BPD. Other studies have associated BPD with wake-sleep cycle disorders.

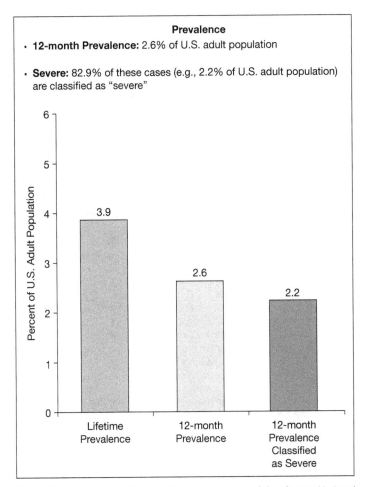

Figure 6.3 Prevalence of bipolar disorders among adults. *Source: National Institute of Mental Health (2016).*

RECOGNIZING SIGNS AND SYMPTOMS OF BIPOLAR DISORDER

ICD-10 Definitions

■ *Bipolar 1 disorder—ICD-10 code F31.60-31.9 definition:* This is a serious, chronic, mood disorder that has characteristic changes in affect, from depression to mania, with periods of remission between recurring episodes. In addition to routine happy and sad periods, people with this disorder intermittently experience extreme emotions, over which they have no control. When experiencing mania, the happy feeling is intense, interfering with activities of daily living. Hopelessness and other feelings that are identified with clinical depression accompanies the depressive episodes. The causes of bipolar disorder are

Table 6.3

Symptoms of Bipolar Disorder

Mania	Hypomania	Depression in bipolar disorder
Symptoms the nurse might see:	*Symptoms the nurse might see:*	*Symptoms the nurse might see:*
■ Energetic, elated, talkative, agitated, pressured speech ■ Believes in an ability to do many things well at the same time ■ Grandiose thinking ■ Sexually reckless ■ May be quick to anger; interferes with socialization ■ May have psychotic features (paranoia, delusions, hallucinations)	■ Much of the same symptoms of mania including mood elevation and energy, with two important differences: 　■ Hypomania does not interfere with work or socialization. 　■ Hypomania does not have psychotic features, and does not require hospitalization. ■ Lasts at least 4 days and is not the patient's usual mood	■ Long periods of sadness ■ Frequent crying spells ■ Changes in sleep and eating patterns ■ Pessimism, anhedonia, guilt, and worry ■ Loss of concentration ■ Physical pains and aches ■ Thoughts of death and suicide
Symptoms the patient will express:	*Symptoms the patient will express:*	*Symptoms the patient will express:*
■ Being "wired," capable of doing amazing things ■ Very jumpy ■ Not needing sleep or to eat or drink ■ Hypersexuality	■ Feeling great ■ No need to sleep ■ Increased impulsive behavior	■ No future; no ability to be happy ever ■ Wishes for death ■ Can't do anything right, worried about ruining everyone's life ■ Tired all the time

not clearly identified, however, anatomy and physiology of the brain are considered have some responsibility, and there is a familial component. Diagnosis of BPD can occur in the teenage years, however BPD is found in children as well as adults.

- *Bipolar II disorder—ICD-10 code F31.81 definition:* Presence of one or more major depressive episodes and at least one episode of hypomania (symptoms that are not as critical as those seen in mania).
- *Cyclothymic disorder (cyclothymia)—ICD-10 F34.0 definition:* This disorder is similar to bipolar disorder, but not as severe. Persons with cyclothymia experience chronic low grade depression alternating with hypomania, over a two year or more period and are at a high risk for developing bipolar disease.

Many people with BPD seek help only when they are depressed, so taking a good history is imperative for adequate treatment. Presenting symptoms are categorized according to seriousness from mild to severe (see Table 6.3).

MEDICATIONS USED TO TREAT BIPOLAR AND RELATED MOOD DISORDERS

A wide range of mood-altering agents are available for use in treating patients with BPD and related mood disorders. They include:

- *Mood stabilizers:* Lithium
- *Anticonvulsants/mood stabilizers*
  - Carbamazepine (Carbatrol, Epitol, Equetro, Tegratol)
  - Divalproex (Depakote)
  - Lamotrigine (Lamictal)
  - Valproic acid (Depakene)
- *Some antipsychotics*
  - Haloperidol (Haldol)
  - Quetiapine Fumarate (Seroquel)
  - Ziprasidone (Geodon)
  - Loxapine (Loxitane)
  - Inhaled loxapine (Adasuve)
  - Risperidone (Risperdal)

THERAPEUTIC AND ENVIRONMENTAL STRATEGIES USED TO TREAT BIPOLAR AND RELATED MOOD DISORDERS

Psychosocial Interventions and Psychotherapy

- *CBT* (see earlier discussion of MDD)
- *Dialectal behavior therapy (DBT)* is an evidence-based therapy that focuses on impulsivity, emotional dysregulation, interpersonal problems, self-harm, and suicidal behaviors. This therapy is comprehensive and helps the person to cope and tolerate distressing events; make treatment plans; reduce counterproductive, dysfunctional behaviors; improve motivation; and adapt to a structured environment (Chapman, 2006).
- *Family-focused therapy* is a solution-focused, time-limited modular therapeutic intervention that teaches the family and the person with BPD communication training and problem solving. It combines psychoeducation and family talk therapy (Morris, Miklowitz, & Waxmonsky, 2007).
- *Psychoeducation* increases illness awareness, self- management skills, habit regularity, and recognition of early warning signs of relapse (Colom, 2014).
- *ECT* (see earlier discussion of MDD)

Environmental Ecotherapies and Strategies

No evidence-based environmental or alternative strategies have been reported that reduce the symptoms of BPD. However, yoga and other naturopathic approaches suggested for patients with MDD are also recommended for those with the depressive symptoms of BPD. Participation in self-help groups is also suggested.

MATCHING NURSING DIAGNOSIS AND MEDICAL DIAGNOSIS

Table 6.4 correlates nursing diagnoses with the ICD-10 codes for bipolar and related disorders.

Table 6.4

Nursing Diagnoses and ICD-10 Nomenclature for Bipolar and Related Disorders	
Nursing diagnoses	**ICD-10 codes**
Risk for violence	Bipolar I disorder (F31.60)
Alteration in coping	Bipolar II disorder (F31.81)
Disturbed thought process	Cyclothymic disorder (cyclothymia; F34.0)
Disturbed sensory perception	
Self-care deficits	

Sources: Herdman & NANDA (2012); ICD10Data.com (n.d.).

SPOTLIGHT ON THE UNIT: YOUNG WOMAN IN THE COMMUNITY CLINIC

Happy, a 36-year-old divorced woman with two children, comes into the community clinic because of a possible sexually transmitted infection. She has been depressed since her divorce 2 years ago, which she initiated because she had fallen in love with another man and didn't feel her husband was good enough for her. She has since been in multiple relationships, each one ending due to her infidelity, or her accusations of infidelity on the part of her partner. Today, Happy appears to be very energetic, even more so than usual. She does not have her children with her, and when asked she says "Oh, I left them with one of my cousins a few days ago. They are such pains...." She is very jumpy and says that she thinks she is pregnant, but if she is, she is sure that it is a girl because she has not had a bite to eat for 4 days and isn't in the least bit hungry or thirsty. When you ask her when she last slept, she laughs very loudly and shouts, "Only jerks need sleep! I have been at the casino, I'm going to win a million dollars and fly away from this place!"

- What are the possible problems you are facing?
- What is the differential diagnosis?

(continued)

- What are the nursing diagnoses?
- To whom should Happy be referred?
- What are your thoughts as to the needs of this family, especially her children?
- What do you do next?

Further Reading

American Psychiatric Association. (2013). *Diagnostic and statistical manual of mental disorders* (5th ed.). Arlington, VA: American Psychiatric Publishing.

Buck, C. (2015, August). *2016 ICD-10: Professional edition.* New York, NY: Saunders.

Leahy, L. G., & Kohler, C. G. (2013). *Manual of clinical psychopharmacology for nurses.* Washington, DC: American Psychiatric Publishing.

National Institute of Mental Health. (2016). Bipolar disorder. Retrieved from https://www.nimh.nih.gov/health/topics/bipolar-disorder/index.shtml

Pilkington, K., Kirkwood, G., Rampes, H., & Richardson, J. (2005, December). Yoga for depression: The research evidence. *Journal of Affective Disorders, 89*(1–3), 13–24.

References

Ahmedani, B. K. (2015, May). Racial/ethnic differences in health care visits made before suicide attempt across the United States. *Medical Care, 53*(5), 430–435.

American Academy of Professional Coders. (n.d.). ICD-10 resource: Coding for major depressive disorder. Retrieved from https://aapcmarketing.s3.amazonaws.com/documents/Depressive-Disorder-ICD-10-BH.pdf

American Psychological Association. (2017). Data on behavioral health in the United States. Retrieved from https://www.apa.org/helpcenter/data-behavioral-health.aspx

Centers for Disease Control and Prevention. (2013). Web-Based Injury Statistics Query and Reporting System (WISQARS) [Online]. Retrieved from http://www.cdc.gov/injury/wisqars/index.html

Chapman, A. L. (2006). Dialectical behavior therapy: Current indications and unique elements. *Psychiatry, 3*(9), 62–68.

Colom, F. (2014). The evolution of psychoeducation for bipolar disorder: From lithium clinics to integrative psychoeducation. *World Psychiatry, 13*(1), 90–92. doi:10.1002/wps.20091

Harvard Health Publications. (2009, April). Yoga for anxiety and depression. Retrieved from http://www.health.harvard.edu/mind-and-mood/yoga-for-anxiety-and-depression

Herdman, T. H., & North American Nursing Diagnosis Association. (2012). *Nursing diagnoses: Definitions & classification 2012–2014.* Chichester, United Kingdom: Wiley-Blackwell.

ICD10Data.com. (n.d.). Retrieved from http://www.icd10data.com

Kessler, R. C., Berglund, P. A., Demler, O., Jin, R., Merikangas, K. R., & Walters, E. E. (2005). Lifetime prevalence and age-of-onset distributions of DSM-IV disorders in the National Comorbidity Survey Replication. *Archives of General Psychiatry, 62*(6), 593–602.

Morris, C. D., Miklowitz, D. J., & Waxmonsky, J. A. (2007). Family-focused treatment for bipolar disorder in adults and youth. *Journal of Clinical Psychology, 63*(5), 433–445. doi:10.1002/jclp.20359

National Institute of Mental Health. (n.d.). Any mood disorder among adults. Retrieved from https://www.nimh.nih.gov/health/statistics/prevalence/any-mood-disorder-among-adults.shtml

National Institute of Mental Health. (2016). Bipolar disorder among adults. Retrieved from http://www.nimh.nih.gov/health/statistics/prevalence/bipolar-disorder-among-adults.shtml

Pratt, L. A., & Brody, D. J. (2014). Depression in the U.S. household population, 2009–2012. NCHS data brief no. 172. Hyattsville, MD: National Center for Health Statistics. Retrieved from https://www.cdc.gov/nchs/data/databriefs/db172.htm

7

Anxiety Disorders

In this chapter, you will learn:

- Statistics related to anxiety disorders
- Neurobiology of anxiety
- How to recognize the signs and symptoms of anxiety disorders
- Prevalent specific anxiety disorders
- Evaluation of presenting symptoms in patients with anxiety disorders
- Common medications and therapeutic strategies used to treat anxiety disorders
- Nursing diagnoses and the *International Classification of Diseases and Related Health Problems*, 10th revision (ICD-10) classifications for anxiety disorders

STATISTICS

The most common of all mental illnesses, anxiety disorders affect approximately 18% of the U.S. population (more than 40 million people). The average age of symptom presentation is 11 years. A number of the anxiety disorders, if not treated in childhood, will persist into adulthood (see Figure 7.1). Anxiety disorder is more common in females (2:1 ratio; American Psychiatric Association, 2013).

It is not unusual for people with anxiety disorder to have other co-morbid mental illnesses. Almost 50% of those diagnosed with an anxiety disorder are also diagnosed with depression. Anxiety disorders

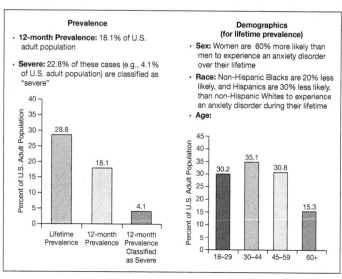

Figure 7.1 Prevalence of any anxiety disorder among adults. *Source: National Institute of Mental Health (n.d.).*

are not outcomes of other physiological illnesses or substance use, although anxiety may be a common symptom of those other disorders. The National Institute of Mental Health (NIMH) identifies several types of anxiety disorders, including generalized anxiety disorder, panic disorder, and social anxiety disorder.

OVERVIEW OF ANXIETY DISORDERS

There are three significant features to observe for when working with a person diagnosed with an anxiety disorder: (a) excessive fear, (b) overwhelming anxiety, and (c) maladaptive behaviors. Anxiety itself is not a psychiatric diagnosis; in fact, it can be very helpful in motivating people to get things done on time. A problem occurs when anxiety becomes persistent and so excessive that daily living is affected. Individuals often feel so overwhelmed by the fear and anxiety that they are unable to work, socialize, or even seek help.

Another word that is often used interchangeably with anxiety is "phobia." Phobias are irrational fears that are specific to a situation (e.g., heights or closed spaces) or objects (e.g., needles or bacteria). Although this chapter focuses on anxiety, rather than the multiple phobias, some of the behavioral components that individuals with anxiety disorders develop to help reduce the anxiety produced by a phobia (e.g., excessive hand washing) are discussed.

Fast Facts in the Spotlight

Anxiety is not pathological unless it interferes with the ability to carry out activities of daily living. It is identified with *excessive* worries and fears. When experienced in our daily lives, anxiety can be an appropriate response, helping us evaluate immediate threats or long-term consequences. Whereas fear is our short-term response to a specific perceived threat, anxiety is the response we have after an event or in anticipation of it. All anxiety disorders share symptoms of co-existing anxiety and fear.

NEUROBIOLOGY OF ANXIETY

Anxiety can result when a neurotransmitter, neuroendocrine, or neuroanatomical disruption in the brain shifts the neuronal activation from the prefrontal cortex, where most executive functioning occurs, to the emotion-regulating limbic system. This increases the likelihood of more visceral responses, denying the ability of the rational executive branch of the brain to evaluate and mitigate stress responses. Neuroimaging, using magnetic resonance imaging (MRI) and functional magnetic imaging (fMRI), has identified hyper-responsiveness to stimuli in the amygdala (the fear center of the brain) in patients diagnosed with anxiety, panic disorder, and posttraumatic stress disorder (Martin, Ressler, Binder, & Nemeroff, 2009). It appears that the brain of a person with an anxiety disorder has encoded the person's responses to stimuli, which block the ability of the higher cognitive part of the brain to repress the negative responses. Patients with generalized anxiety disorder have been found to have increased amygdala volume.

If a person is unable to access the prefrontal cortex because of severe, persistent anxiety, it is as though he or she has been emotionally hijacked. During those times, the patient cannot relax, self-soothe, or process any environmental cues being provided. These patients are in a state of total emotional dysfunction.

Serotonin and Anxiety

Changes in the levels of serotonin, a neurotransmitter in the brain, influence both mood and behavior. Three models have been theorized to explain the link between serotonin and anxiety: (a) the see-saw model, (b) the amygdala model, and (c) the basal ganglia model (Stein & Stahl, 2000). In all three models, the inability to regulate serotonin during anxiety is a central feature, resulting in an inability to mitigate the fear response. Stein and Stahl (2000) emphasize that the intricacies and complexities of anxiety and brain function cannot be easily explained by models; however, these models provide some guidance for researchers developing medications to mitigate the debilitating effects of anxiety disorders.

RECOGNIZING SIGNS AND SYMPTOMS OF ANXIETY DISORDERS

The presenting symptoms of anxiety disorders are sweating, trembling, chest pain, shortness of breath, and heart palpitations. Patients may say that it feels as though nothing is real, express a fear of dying, and be hypervigilant, seeking a way to escape. Frequently patients experience tingling in the limbs, become flushed, or complain of chills. Their ability to respond to everyday questions may be affected, and their response to the possibility of environmental danger heightened. A patient may have had insomnia in the preceding days, have some difficulty swallowing because of dry mouth, have numbness in the hands or feet, or be very fidgety.

Fast Facts in the Spotlight

Anxiety may be associated with heart disease and risk factors for heart attack (McCann, n.d.). People with anxiety disorders may experience tachycardia, hypertension, and decreased heart rate variability. Because 50% of people with depression also have an anxiety disorder, and depression has been linked to coronary heart disease, it is important to examine the patient with anxiety for any heart problems.

PREVALENT SPECIFIC ANXIETY DISORDERS

Specific Phobias

Specific phobias are defined as persistent fear of objects or situations that result in immediate extreme anxiety. Behavioral alterations reflect a desire to avoid the object or situation at all costs, demonstrating an uncontrollable, irrational response. This response has a negative effect on other areas of living, such as employment, social attachments, and activities of daily living. Children and adolescents may react with varying degrees of freezing, crying, acting out, or holding onto the caregiver.

Social Anxiety Disorder

Social anxiety disorder is diagnosed when an individual demonstrates a persistent (for at least 6 months) extreme fear of being negatively evaluated by others in social situations. The fear extends to worrying about engaging in actions that will be humiliating. The individual attempts to change behaviors to avoid the social situations completely; if that is not possible, he or she is forced to experience them while feeling an overwhelming sense of anxiety and worry. Onset of symptoms is usually between the ages of 8 and 15 years. Children and adolescents experience this disorder with peers and in adult social situations, and they may respond by throwing tantrums and refusing to participate in activities.

Generalized Anxiety Disorder

In adults, generalized anxiety disorder is defined as excessive and persistent worrying and feelings of anxiety over a period of 6 months or more, such that the level of worry and anxiety has significantly interfered with work, socializing, or daily functioning. The ongoing experience results in a sense of fatigue, difficulty concentrating, disturbances in sleep patterns, and muscle tension. The mean age of onset for generalized anxiety disorder is about 30 years.

Panic Disorder

Panic disorder is an intense, paralyzing apprehension accompanied by a sense of impending doom, which produces physical effects such as shortness of breath, a sense of choking, chest pain, and palpitations.

These symptoms occur without warning and not in response to any specific known environmental or emotional stimuli. A panic attack is usually of short duration, but in rare instances it may be prolonged. Patients who have panic disorder are often apprehensive about the possibility of experiencing an attack and frequently alter their behavior in an attempt to avoid one. These patients have an increased rate of suicide.

Anxiety Symptoms Secondary to an Existing Medical Condition

Medical conditions that may be an underlying cause of panic or anxiety in a patient include:

- *Endocrine disorders*: Hyperthyroidism, hypoglycemia, and hyperadrenocortisolism
- *Respiratory disorders:* Asthma, chronic obstructive pulmonary disease, pneumonia
- *Cardiovascular disorders:* Emboli, atrial fibrillation, congestive heart failure
- *Neurological disorders:* Seizure disorder, neoplasms, encephalitis
- *Vitamin deficiencies:* Vitamin B_{12} deficiency

Anxiety Secondary to Substance Use

This category applies when a patient presents with anxiety that is secondary to use of or withdrawal from a substance, and the excessive anxiety experienced is the factor having the impact on functioning.

Postpartum Anxiety

Although postpartum depression is a well-known disorder affecting new mothers, women may also develop postpartum anxiety, which is an apprehension of death and danger after childbirth, leading to specific avoidance-prone behaviors that are disabling or interfere with activities of daily living.

MEDICATIONS USED TO TREAT ANXIETY DISORDERS

Many different medications are available for the treatment of anxiety disorders. Categories of medications are listed in Table 7.1.

Table 7.1

Categories of Medications Commonly Used for Anxiety Disorders

Category	Generic name	Brand name(s)
Benzodiazepines	alprazolam	Xanax
	clonazepam	Klonopin
	diazepam	Valium
	lorazepam	Ativan
Beta-blockers	metoprolol	Lopressor
	metoprolol LX	Toprol-LX
	propranolol	Inderal
	atenolol	Tenormin
Tricyclic antidepressants (TCAs)	doxepin	Sinequan
	clomipramine HCl	Anafranil
	imipramine	Tofranil
Other antidepressants	bupropion	Wellbutrin
	amitriptyline (tricyclic)	Amitid, Amitril, Elavil
	nortriptyline (tricyclic)	Pamelor
Monoamine oxidase inhibitors (MAOIs)	isocarboxazid	Marplan
	phenelzine	Nardil
	tranylcypromine	Parnate
	selegiline	Emsam
Selective serotonin reuptake inhibitors (SSRIs)	sertraline	Zoloft
	fluoxetine	Prozac
	escitalopram	Lexapro
	citalopram	Celexa
	paroxetine	Paxil
	fluvoxamine	Luvox
Serotonin–norepinephrine reuptake inhibitors (SNRIs)	desvenlafaxine	Pristiq
	duloxetine	Cymbalta
	venlafaxine	Effexor XR
Mild tranquilizers	buspirone	BuSpar
Anticonvulsants	quetiapine	Seroquel

THERAPEUTIC AND ENVIRONMENTAL STRATEGIES USED TO TREAT ANXIETY DISORDERS

Psychosocial Interventions and Psychotherapy

Several different psychotherapies have been demonstrated to be effective in treating anxiety disorders.

- *Cognitive behavioral therapy (CBT)* is often used in conjunction with pharmacotherapy with good effect.
- *Exposure therapy* is a form of CBT in which the person is exposed to the feared solution, allowing the brain to adapt to the experience of anxiety during the introduction of the stimuli. There are four general variations of exposure therapy: (a) in vivo (direct confrontation of the fear object), (b) imaginal (imagining the feared object), (c) virtual (digital reconstruction of the feared object; e.g., online driving of a car in virtual traffic), and (d) interoceptive (creating a physical sensation and learning how to deal with it; e.g., tachycardia after exercising). Pacing of the exposure therapy is also important. Interventions can be paced as graded exposure (starts with mild experiences and progresses to more difficult ones), flooding (starts with the hardest experience), or systematic desensitization (often combined with relaxation so that the focus of fear becomes associated with relaxing).
- *Sensorimotor psychotherapy* is a form of somatic therapy that uses therapeutic interactivity to facilitate regulation of a client's dysregulated emotional response. It is a body-based talk therapy that involves mindfulness, collaboration, and client self-awareness of body sensations.

Therapeutic Techniques

Nurses without formal training in these therapeutic techniques can rely on therapeutic alliance skills to support the person with an anxiety disorder.

- *"Listen, believe, empathize"*: Anxiety is a brain disorder. Your patient has come for help. Listen with respect and believe that what your patient is telling you is real to the patient. Ask your patient what has worked in the past to reduce the anxiety. If possible, incorporate the patient's suggestions into the care plan.

Table 7.2

Nursing Diagnosis and ICD-10 Nomenclature for Anxiety Disorders	
Nursing diagnoses	**ICD-10 codes**
Anxiety	Anxiety disorder, unspecified (F41.9)
Fear	Generalized anxiety (F41.1)
Real or perceived threat of (1) death, (2) self-concept	Panic disorder (F41.0)
Ineffective coping	(Each anxiety disorder has its own ICD-10 code)
Ineffective impulse control	

Sources: Herdman & NANDA (2012); ICD10Data.com (n.d.).

- *Reduce environmental stimuli:* Where possible, reduce the noise, lights, and normal commotion that are common in many areas of patient treatment centers. Ask the patient if the changes you are making are reducing the sense of worry.

MATCHING NURSING DIAGNOSIS AND MEDICAL DIAGNOSIS

Table 7.2 correlates nursing diagnoses with the *International Statistical Classification of Diseases and Related Health Problems*, 10th revision (ICD-10) codes for anxiety disorders.

SPOTLIGHT ON THE UNIT: WOMAN WITH PANIC DISORDER IN THE POSTANESTHESIA CARE UNIT (PACU)

Mrs. Z is a middle-aged woman who was admitted this morning for foot surgery. When she met with you before surgery, she reported that she was a highly anxious person and had been taking clonazepam (Klonopin), 1 mg three times a day, for the past 20 years. Some days she took the medication only in the morning and at night, skipping the midday dose. She has not taken any pills since 9 p.m. the night before.

(continued)

As she is awakening from anesthesia in the PACU, she starts to fidget with the sheets. She calls out "Nurse! Nurse! Oh my God, I think I'm going to die!" You notice that her blood pressure is going up. Whereas it had been 110/70 mm Hg on admission and 110/82 post-operatively, it is now 150/90. Her pulse is 92 bpm and her respirations are very rapid and shallow at 26/min. As you approach the bed, she is crying and shaking, and tells you she is so scared that her chest hurts and she can't breathe. The pulse oximetry reading is 98%.

- What are the possible problems you are facing?
- What differential diagnosis might you consider?
- What are the nursing diagnoses?
- Whom should you call to assess Mrs. Z in the PACU?
- What are your thoughts about the needs of this patient, during hospitalization and after?
- What kind of hand-off report might you need to give to the floor nurses?
- What do you do next?

Further Reading

American Psychological Association. (n.d.). What is exposure therapy? Retrieved from http://www.div12.org/sites/default/files/WhatIsExposure Therapy.pdf

Anxiety and Depression Association of America. (n.d.). Symptoms. Retrieved from https://www.ADAA.org/understanding-anxiety/specific-phobias/symptoms

Buck, C. (2015, August). *2016 ICD-10: Professional edition*. New York, NY: Saunders.

LeBano, L. (2013). The circuitry of fear: Understanding the neurobiology of PTSD. Retrieved from http://www.psychcongress.com/article/circuitry-fear-understanding-neurobiology-ptsd-13639

Halter, M. J., & Varcarolis, E. M. (2014). *Varcarolis' foundations of psychiatric mental health nursing: A clinical approach*. St. Louis, MO: Elsevier.

Nussbaum, A. (2013). *The pocket guide to the DSM-5 diagnostic exam*. Arlington, VA: American Psychiatric Publishing.

Stahl, S., & Grady, M. (2010). *Stahl's illustrated anxiety, stress, and PTSD*. Boston, MA: Cambridge University Press.

References

American Psychiatric Association. (2013). *Diagnostic and statistical manual of mental disorders* (5th ed.). Arlington, VA: American Psychiatric Publishing.

Herdman, T. H., & North American Nursing Diagnosis Association. (2012). *Nursing diagnoses: Definitions & classification 2012–2014*. Chichester, United Kingdom: Wiley-Blackwell.

ICD10Data.com. (n.d.). Retrieved from http://www.icd10data.com

Martin, D., Ressler, K., Binder, E., & Nemeroff, C. (2009). The neurobiology of anxiety disorders: Brain imaging, genetics and psychoneuroendocrinology. *The Psychiatric Clinics of North America*, *32*(3), 549–575.

McCann, U. (n.d.). Anxiety and heart disease. Heart & Vascular Institute, Johns Hopkins Medicine. Retrieved from http://www.hopkinsmedicine.org/heart_vascular_institute/clinical_services

National Institute of Mental Health. (n.d.). Any anxiety disorder among adults. Retrieved from http://www.nimh.nih.gov/health/statistics/prevalence/any-anxiety-disorder-among-adults.shtml

Stein, D., & Stahl, S. (2000). Serotonin and anxiety: Current models. *International Clinical Psychopharmacology*, *15*(Suppl. 2), S1–S6.

8

Obsessive Compulsive Disorder and Related Disorders

In this chapter, you will learn:

- Statistics related to obsessive compulsive disorder (OCD) and related disorders
- How to recognize the signs and symptoms of OCD
- Prevalent specific related disorders
- Common medications and therapeutic strategies used to treat OCD
- Nursing diagnoses and the *International Classification of Diseases and Related Health Problems*, 10th revision (ICD-10) classifications for OCD and related disorders

STATISTICS

OCD affects slightly more than 1% of Americans (see Figure 8.1). Men are more often diagnosed in childhood and women more often in adulthood. The average age at onset of symptoms is 19 years, but it is not unusual to observe OCD in boys younger than 10 years of age. Children who are negative and internalize their feelings are at a higher risk for developing OCD. Symptoms usually develop over time.

Forty percent of patients diagnosed with OCD in childhood or adolescence usually experience remission of the disease in early

Demographics
(for lifetime prevalence)

- **Sex:** Not Reported
- **Race:** Not Reported
- **Age:**

Prevalence

- **12-month Prevalence:** 1.0% of U.S. adult population
- **Severe:** 50.6% of these cases (e.g., 0.5% of U.S. adult population) are classified as "severe"

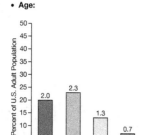

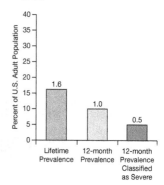

Figure 8.1 Obsessive compulsive disorder among adults. *Source: National Institute of Mental Health (n.d.).*

adulthood (American Psychiatric Association, 2013). Like patients with other psychiatric diagnoses, those with OCD may have comorbid psychiatric diagnoses, such as anxiety disorder, phobias, depression, or bipolar disease. These comorbidities increase the risk for suicide ideation and attempts.

OVERVIEW OF OCD

OCD is characterized by obsessions and compulsions. *Obsessions* are thoughts, urges, or images that persistently and repeatedly occur to an individual. The intrusive thoughts, urges, or images cause anxiety that interferes with daily living. *Compulsions* are uncontrollable, persistent, repetitive behaviors, often evolving within a rule-guided framework to avoid or control the obsessions. The behaviors, however, are unrealistic and also interfere with the patient's ability to engage in daily activities at work, home, and in the community.

Psychopathologies related to OCD are hoarding disorder, hair-pulling disorder (trichotillomania), and skin-picking disorder (excoriation). These disorders reflect a compulsive action that is used to decrease the person's high level of anxiety. Patients do not have any control over these behaviors, and despite negative outcomes and repeated attempts to stop, they are unable to do so.

RECOGNIZING SIGNS AND SYMPTOMS OF OCD

The presenting symptoms of OCD are persistent intrusive thoughts (obsessions) that are believed to be reduced through the engagement of repetitive behaviors (compulsions). The thoughts and behaviors take up a lot of the patient's time and interfere with normal activities of daily living. The thoughts are intrusive, unwanted, and without pleasure. The behaviors are considered to be compulsions when they are repetitive, excessive, bound by rigid rules, used to reduce the thoughts that are fueling the anxiety, and not actually connected in any realistic way to the anxiety-provoking thought.

Themes that have emerged related to the obsessions and compulsions include contamination, symmetry, harm, and unwanted thoughts. Situations can trigger the obsession or compulsion, or both.

Fast Facts in the Spotlight

Children who have experienced trauma (including physical or sexual abuse) are at higher risk of OCD, as are those with a first-degree relative with the disorder. No one culture demonstrates a higher incidence of OCD, and across all cultures the same themes appear.

PREVALENT SPECIFIC RELATED DISORDERS

Body Dysmorphic Disorder

Body dysmorphic disorder is reflected in obsessions with one's appearance, specifically with flaws or perceived defects. It occurs in slightly more than 2% of adults in the United States and is most commonly observed in patients seeking the advice of dermatologists, cosmetic surgeons, and oral surgeons.

Hoarding Disorders

Hoarding disorder is identified in people who have extreme behavior involving acquisition of or difficulty discarding possessions. Over time this causes the individual's home environment to become unusable and unhealthy. Significant hoarding is seen in about 2% to 6% of the global population, and it is more prevalent in older adults.

Body-Related Psychopathologies

- *Trichotillomania*, or hair pulling, is expressed as the need to pull hairs out of one's own body with an inability to stop, despite the despair it causes.
- *Excoriation disorder*, or skin picking, occurs despite the person's desire to stop. It results in the development of scabs and causes increased emotional distress.

Substance-Induced OCD-Like Disorders

Substance-induced OCD-like disorders are seen in conjunction with a person's use of an intoxicating medication (e.g., methamphetamine or other stimulant).

MEDICATIONS USED TO TREAT OCD

The medications most commonly used to treat OCD are antidepressants, among them:

- Clomipramine (Anafranil)
- Fluoxetine (Prozac)
- Fluvoxamine (Luvox)
- Paroxetine (Paxil, Pexeva)
- Sertraline (Zoloft)

THERAPEUTIC AND ENVIRONMENTAL STRATEGIES USED TO TREAT OCD

Psychosocial Interventions and Psychotherapy

Psychotherapy focuses on assisting the patient to control his or her OCD.

- *Cognitive behavioral therapy (CBT)* is a goal-oriented approach to problem solving that uses therapy supported by homework assignments, which change patterned thinking, behaviors, or both.

- *Mindfulness therapy* supports the patient to remain aware of the present moment, refrain from passing judgment, and accept the discomfort associated with certain thoughts.

Environmental Strategies

- *Exposure and response prevention (ERP) therapy* provides gradual exposure to the item that is feared or repulsed. It requires time and practice but can support the patient in getting used to dealing with the stimulus that triggers the OCD response (e.g., dirt).
- The Yale–Brown Obsessive Compulsive Scale (YBOCS) can help identify the symptoms present in a person with OCD and can be used to assist the therapist in developing the ERP therapy.

MATCHING NURSING DIAGNOSIS AND MEDICAL DIAGNOSIS

Table 8.1 correlates nursing diagnoses with the ICD-10 codes for OCD and related disorders.

Table 8.1

Nursing Diagnosis and ICD-10 Nomenclature for OCD and Related Disorders	
Nursing diagnoses	**ICD-10 codes**
Ineffective coping	Obsessive compulsive disorder (OCD; F42)
Ineffective impulse control	
Disturbed body image	Hoarding disorder (F42.3)
	Excoriation disorder (F42.4)
	Other OCD (F42.8)
	OCD, unspecified (F42.9)

Sources: Herdman & NANDA (2012); ICD10Data.com (n.d.).

SPOTLIGHT ON THE UNIT: GRADUATE NURSING STUDENT WITH RITUAL BEHAVIORS

Nurse L is a graduate nursing student who was known to friends and colleagues as the most fastidious of the unit nurses. When preparing the procedure room for a patient, she engaged in a number of rituals, measuring tape, lining up items to be used, and arranging the room so that nothing was even a millimeter out of order. Nurse L's obsession with cleanliness began to increase, often interfering with the unit's ability to get patients in and out of the room in a timely manner. Nurse L was seeing a therapist, but never told the therapist about the need to keep everything controlled and clean because of a fear of being labeled "nutty." On several particularly busy days, Nurse L's obsessions and compulsions disrupted the unit's ability to meet all of the patients' needs, resulting in her dismissal from the unit.

Subsequently Nurse L presents to the school clinic. She complains of being depressed, not eating at all, and sleeping for hours each day. When not sleeping, Nurse L is using tape to line up the magazines and other items on the tables in her apartment. Issues such as handwashing have now caused scars and rashes on her hands. Nurse L is embarrassed about the situation.

- What are the possible problems you are facing?
- What are the nursing diagnoses?
- What are your thoughts about the needs of this patient?
- What do you do?

Further Reading

American Psychiatric Association. (2015). What is a hoarding disorder? Retrieved from https://www.psychiatry.org/patients-families/hoarding-disorder/what-is-hoarding-disorder

Wahl, K., Huelle, J. Zurowski, B., & Kordon, A. (2012). Managing obsessive thoughts during brief exposure: An experimental study comparing mindfulness-based strategies and distraction in obsessive-compulsive disorder. *Cognitive Therapy and Research*, *37*(4), 752–761. doi:10.1007/s10608-012-9503-2

References

American Psychiatric Association. (2013). *Diagnostic and statistical manual of mental disorders* (5th ed.). Arlington, VA: American Psychiatric Publishing.

Herdman, T. H., & North American Nursing Diagnosis Association. (2012). *Nursing diagnoses: Definitions & classification 2012–2014*. Chichester, United Kingdom: Wiley-Blackwell.

ICD10Data.com. (n.d.). Retrieved from http://www.icd10data.com

National Institute of Mental Health. (n.d.). Obsessive compulsive disorder among adults. Retrieved from http://www.nimh.nih.gov/health/statistics/prevalence/obsessive-compulsive-disorder-among-adults.shtml

9

Trauma and Stress: Posttraumatic Stress Disorder and Related Disorders

In this chapter, you will learn:

- Statistics related to posttraumatic stress disorder (PTSD) and other related disorders
- Neurobiology of PTSD
- How to recognize the signs and symptoms of PTSD
- Prevalent specific related disorders
- Common medications and therapeutic strategies used to treat PTSD
- Nursing diagnoses and the *International Classification of Diseases*, 10th revision (ICD-10) classifications for PTSD and related disorders

STATISTICS

PTSD occurs in about 3.5% of the U.S. adult population and has an average age of onset of 23 years (see Figure 9.1). Between 15% and 25% of military veterans experience PTSD. The disorder includes a spectrum of psychoemotional as well as physiopathological responses and outcomes.

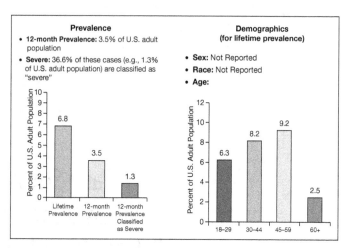

Figure 9.1 Prevalence and demographics of PTSD among adults.
Source: National Institute of Mental Health (n.d.).

OVERVIEW OF PTSD

PTSD is a complicated disorder that includes a cornucopia of symptoms ranging from changes in ability to feel safe to engaging in self-injurious behaviors. The National Institute for Mental Health (NIMH) defines PTSD as an anxiety disorder experienced after an individual is exposed to an event in which his or her own life or the life of a loved one is exposed to dire physical harm. This event can be real, such as war, or perceived, such as watching a terror attack on television. The symptoms of PTSD may occur soon after the event or years later. What is common in both scenarios is that the individual feels the horror, helplessness, and intense fear of the event. The person who has PTSD carries the persistent fear and stress of the danger, re-experiencing arousal with reactive symptoms, even when the danger has passed.

PTSD can be acute (short term) or chronic (long term), and the effects interfere with activities of daily living, such as employment and relationships. The recurrent memories (flashbacks) may result in dissociation, withdrawal, depression, and amnesia. People who have PTSD are often unpredictable when stressed and can react with aggression, recklessness, or self-injurious behaviors. Children younger than 6 years of age who experience PTSD may become overly attached to their caretaker, stop speaking, begin bedwetting, or play-act the event.

Disorders that are related to PTSD include acute stress disorder, reactive attachment disorder, disinhibited social engagement disorder, and adjustment disorders. The ICD-10 places PTSD under the category of Reaction to Severe Stress (F43) (see Table 9.1, later in this chapter).

NEUROBIOLOGY OF PTSD

The parts of the brain that respond to stress—the amygdala, hippocampus, and prefrontal cortex—are all important in the diagnosis of PTSD. These critical regions affect the brain's ability to mediate threats. People with PTSD respond to stressors with increased release of cortisol and norepinephrine. PTSD may decrease hippocampal and anterior cingulate volumes. The amygdala (which activates our responses to fight, flight, freeze, or submit) is overactive, while responses from the medial prefrontal cortex (executive function) decrease.

These changes in the brain of a person with PTSD lead to the symptoms of intrusive thoughts. This process is important for understanding the patient's stress response as well as the pharmacological and therapeutic approaches to treating trauma.

RECOGNIZING SIGNS AND SYMPTOMS OF PTSD

Different individuals will exhibit different signs and symptoms of PTSD, depending on the severity of their trauma and the coping mechanisms they have learned to use over time in dealing with their symptoms. This is worth emphasizing. PTSD includes symptoms of other psychiatric disorders (anxiety, depression, and avoidant behaviors); therefore, a thorough history is important for best treatment to rule out other diagnoses. Suicidal ideation, as well as suicide attempts and completions, are high in the PTSD population. This increased potential for suicide may be due to the combination of depression, anxiety, agitation, and poor impulse control. Vigilance in assessing for this possibility is critical.

Common symptoms of PTSD in children and adults are as follows:

- *Children:* Avoidant behaviors, reduction in engagement in social activities, moodiness, and reporting of frightening dreams or nightmares (problems with sleep exist in children of all ages diagnosed with PTSD)

- *Young adults:* Self-depreciating image, sense of cowardice, reluctance to engage in new activities, aggressiveness, and reckless disregard for safety
- *Adults:* Intrusive memories of traumatic events that cause emotional arousal, emotional shutdown, or dissociation

People with PTSD often have exaggerated negative opinions of themselves, are unable to enjoy positive experiences and emotions, and experience myriad symptoms, including hypervigilance. Changes in mood and cognition are common among people who survive a traumatic event and develop PTSD. It is not unusual for a person to be unable to remember the traumatic event; to demonstrate a negative attitude toward self and the future; and to blame himself or herself, or others, for the event, despite the lack of evidence to support that belief.

Fast Facts in the Spotlight

The symptoms of PTSD are thought to present in three ways, which are often referred to as "clusters":

1. The individual with PTSD might *relive* the trauma, either in thoughts or in night/day mares. The physical and emotional response during the reliving experience will be real and present.
2. *Avoidance* of any reminders or triggers is another set of symptoms, causing the individual to withdraw from normal activities of daily living.
3. *Hypervigilance* is the third cluster of symptoms. People with PTSD may have insomnia, irritability, lack of concentration, loss of memories, and be hyper-reactive to noise or unanticipated events.

Evaluating Presenting Symptoms

Symptoms of PTSD can occur as soon as 1 day after experiencing a traumatic event, but may not present until years later. The symptoms that will be noticed by individuals or their family members can include:

- Intrusive, unwanted memories
- Numbed, almost dissociative-like response, to talking about the experience
- Depression
- Survivor's guilt
- Panic attacks
- Nightmares
- Insomnia
- Hyperarousal and hypervigilance

Depression, substance abuse, and self-injurious behaviors may also be present, accompanied by relationship, social, and occupational problems. Patients with PTSD often seem to be "hijacked" by their thoughts and memories, carried back into the past. Consideration of possible comorbidities is essential as pharmaceutical interventions may have either a positive or negative impact on these disorders. Medications alone do not provide the best outcomes for these patients, who require a strong support system and therapeutic interventions to address this complicated diagnosis.

Fast Facts in the Spotlight

PTSD occurs when individuals either experience or are exposed to an event that makes them fear for their life or the lives of those they love. It can occur as a result of war or of watching or experiencing attacks through the television, but may also result from a traumatic event that occurs unexpectedly in an individual's daily life (e.g., a mugging, dog attack, or other violent confrontation). Media coverage of traumatic events may trigger and help maintain an individual's symptoms of PTSD after the event (Hamblin, 2016).

Diagnostic Screening Tools

Many screening tools for PTSD can be found at the National Center for PTSD website (U.S. Department of Veterans Affairs, 2017). They include:

- Chart screens for PTSD
- Beck Anxiety Inventory (BAI-PC)

- Primary Care PTSD Screen (PC-PTSD)
- Short form of the PTSD checklist—civilian version
- Short Screening Scale for PTSD
- Trauma Screening Questionnaire (TSQ)

PREVALENT SPECIFIC RELATED DISORDERS

PTSD is associated with the following psychological disorders:

- *Anxiety disorders* (see Chapter 7).
- *Acute stress reaction*: This disorder is seen *within 1 month* of experiencing an acute traumatic event. The symptoms may include anxiety and some dissociative features. If the symptoms persist for over 1 month, the diagnosis changes to *PTSD*.
- *Adjustment disorder*: A maladaptive response to stressors in which the emotional response begins within 3 months of experiencing the stressor (e.g., loss of a job) and lasts for about 6 months.
- *Psychogenic, nonepileptic seizure (PNES)*: A somatic, involuntary response that is associated with acute or repressed traumatic events of childhood. Presenting symptoms can resemble those seen in partial or generalized seizures, and are commonly first diagnosed by neurologists. PNES is usually seen in patients with previously diagnosed stress disorder or trauma experienced in childhood. These seizures most frequently present in adolescents and adults, and are three times more common in women. The diagnosis of a seizure disorder is ruled out through a comprehensive seizure evaluation in which the electroencephalogram is negative for any aberrant electrical brain activity. (Seizure workup is discussed in detail in Chapter 13.)

MEDICATIONS USED TO TREAT PTSD

Pharmacotherapy focuses on modifying the neurotransmitters that can reduce the fear and anxiety reactions. These neurotransmitters include dopamine, serotonin, gamma-aminobutyric acid (GABA), and N-methyl-D-aspartate (NDMA). Among the varied agents that may be prescribed for patients with PTSD are:

- *Selective serotonin reuptake inhibitors (SSRIs)*: Sertraline (Zoloft), paroxetine (Paxil), and fluoxetine (Prozac)

- *Other antidepressants*: Mirtazapine (Remeron), venlafaxine (Effexor), and nefazodone (Serzone)
- *Mood stabilizers*: Carbamazepine (Tegretol), divalproex (Depakote), lamotrigine (Lamictal), and topiramate (Topamax)
- *Benzodiazepines*: Lorazepam (Ativan), clonazepam (Klonopin), alprazolam (Xanax), and diazepam (Valium)
- *Other medications*: Prazosin (Minipress), clonidine (Catapres), tricyclic antidepressants, and monoamine oxidase inhibitors (MAOIs)

THERAPEUTIC AND ENVIRONMENTAL STRATEGIES USED TO TREAT PTSD

As research continues into best practice for the treatment of PTSD, methods for treatment also evolve. Therapeutic strategies currently used for patients with PTSD are outlined here.

Group and Family Therapies

- *Group therapy*: Sharing the experience with others who have had the same or similar experiences may reduce the shame, guilt, and fear of the diagnosis. Participants build social and therapeutic relationships that support the development of self-worth and trust.
- *Family therapy*: The entire family works with a therapist to improve communication and relationships, and works through the hard moments that arise with compassion and patience.

Individual Therapies

- *Cognitive behavioral therapy (CBT)*: CBT helps patients to identify the thoughts that make them feel distressed and learn ways to cope with the feelings.
- *Prolonged exposure therapy*: Repeatedly talking about the trauma teaches the person not to fear the memory, and develops strategies to cope with the feelings when they arise.
- *Eye movement desensitization and reprocessing (EMDR)*: Following the therapist's hand with eye movements helps to change the way the brain reacts to the memory of the event.
- *Sensorimotor psychotherapy*: This somatic sensing technique is used to process bottom-up emotional states and teaches the person strategies for autoregulation.

Fast Facts in the Spotlight

Predictive factors for PTSD have been identified—factors that make one person more likely to develop the disorder than another who experiences the same trauma. According to Stahl and Grady (2010), strong predictors for developing PTSD after trauma are a psychiatric history, experience of childhood abuse, or a family history of psychiatric problems. Moderate predictors are lack of social supports, prior experience of trauma, having an adverse childhood experience, having life stress, and a very severe traumatic experience. Genetically people with a small hippocampus, those with hypocortisolism, and individuals with genetic polymorphisms may be at risk. The type of trauma experienced should always be taken into account.

MATCHING NURSING DIAGNOSIS AND MEDICAL DIAGNOSIS

Table 9.1 correlates nursing diagnoses with the ICD-10 codes for PTSD and related disorders.

Table 9.1

Nursing Diagnosis and ICD-10 Nomenclature for PTSD	
Nursing diagnoses	**ICD-10 codes**
Posttrauma syndrome: "Sustained maladaptive response to a traumatic, overwhelming event"	Posttraumatic stress disorder (PTSD) (F43.1)
	PTSD unspecified (F43.1)
Anxiety	PTSD, acute (F43.11)
Risk for violence to self or others	PTSD, chronic (F43.12)
Ineffective coping	Acute stress reaction (F43.0)
Risk-prone health behavior	Adjustment disorder (F43.2)

Sources: Herdman & NANDA (2012); ICD10data.com (n.d.).

SPOTLIGHT ON THE UNIT: ADOLESCENT IN THE TRAUMA CENTER

Benji arrived at the trauma center with his friend Robert after both were in a boating accident. Benji, 15 years old, is a good swimmer and pulled Robert (age 13) to shore after their jet skis were hit by a larger boat in the nearby lake. Robert suffered a broken arm, but Benji did not have any visible injuries. As Benji explains what occurred, describing the lake as being very crowded with boats, windsurfers, and jet skiers, he recalls the event "like it's still happening in slow motion." Benji's voice slows and his body goes very still as he remembers, "the boat was coming fast. I yelled at Robert, but he didn't hear. I chased his jet ski, knowing that I was being crazy— that we would both get killed. I got close to Robert's jet ski when suddenly we were both off the skis and flying toward the water. I came back up and saw Robert's jet ski, but not him. I freaked! I swam over the jet ski and found him with his harness attached to the ski . . . his arm all busted and twisted. I called his name but he didn't answer. It was just like a movie—and when my sister got hit by a car. . . ." Suddenly Benji goes very silent and his hand begins to twitch. You call to him, but he doesn't answer, he is crying, but without a sound and not responding to those around him.

- What do you think is happening?
- What can you do?

Further Reading

Adshead, G. (2000). Psychological therapies for post-traumatic stress disorder. *The British Journal of Psychiatry*, *177*(2), 144–148.

Bremner, J. D. (2006). Traumatic stress: Effects on the brain. *Dialogues in Clinical Neuroscience*, *8*(4), 445–461.

Department of Veterans Affairs. (2002). Post traumatic stress disorder: Implications for primary care. Independent study course. Retrieved from https://www.publichealth.va.gov/docs/vhi/posttraumatic.pdf

Gibson, L. (2016). Acute stress disorder. U.S. Department of Veterans Affairs. Retrieved from https://www.ptsd.va.gov/professional/treatment/early/acute-stress-disorder.asp

Iribarren, J., Prolo, P., Neagos, N., & Chiappelli, F. (2005). Post-traumatic stress disorder: Evidence-based research for the third millennium. *Evidence-Based Complementary and Alternative Medicine*, *2*(4), 503–512.

Jeffreys, M. (2017). Clinicians guide to medications for PTSD. Retrieved from
https://www.ptsd.va.gov/professional/treatment/overview/clinicians-guide
-to-medications-for-ptsd.asp

Ogden, P., & Minton, K. (2000, October). Sensori-motor psychotherapy: One
method for processing traumatic memory. *Traumatology, VI*(3). Retrieved
from https://www.sensorimotorpsychotherapy.org/articles.html

References

Hamblin, J. (2016). Media coverage of traumatic events: Research on effects.
Retrieved from http://www.ptsd.va.gov/professional/trauma/basics/media
-coverage-traumatic-events.asp

Herdman, T. H., & North American Nursing Diagnosis Association. (2012).
Nursing diagnoses: Definitions & classification 2012–2014. Chichester,
United Kingdom: Wiley-Blackwell.

ICD10data.com (n.d.). Retrieved from http://www.icd10data.com

National Institute of Mental Health. (n.d.). Post-traumatic stress disorder
among adults. Retrieved from https://www.nimh.nih.gov/health/statistics/
prevalence/post-traumatic-stress-disorder-among-adults.shtml

Stahl, S., & Grady, M. (2010). *Stahl's illustrated anxiety, stress, and PTSD.*
New York, NY: Cambridge University Press.

U.S. Department of Veterans Affairs. (2017). PTSD: National Center for PTSD:
List of all measures. Retrieved from https://www.ptsd.va.gov/professional/
assessment/all_measures.asp

10

Neurocognitive and Neurodegenerative Disorders

In this chapter, you will learn:

- Statistics related to neurocognitive and neurodegenerative disorders
- How to recognize the signs and symptoms of neurocognitive and neurodegenerative disorders
- Evaluation of presenting symptoms in patients with these disorders
- Common medications and therapeutic strategies used to treat neurocognitive and neurodegenerative disorders
- Nursing diagnoses and the *International Classification of Diseases and Related Health Problems*, 10th revision (ICD-10) classifications for these disorders

STATISTICS

Neurocognitive Disorders

The term *neurocognitive disorder* refers to delirium, dementia, amnesic disorders, and other disorders affecting cognitive functions. Alzheimer's disease is the most common disorder causing dementia. Neurocognitive disorders are divided into major neurocognitive disorders (dementias) and mild neurocognitive disorders.

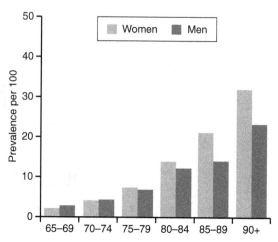

Figure 10.1 Pooled prevalence of dementia by sex, based on Lobo et al. *Source: Data from Lobo et al. (2000).*

A patient with dementia usually has symptoms that have compromised the ability to function in a social or occupational arena. Neurocognitive disorders increase with age (see Figure 10.1). The prevalence of mild cognitive disorder is estimated to be between 2% and 10% in adults at 65 years of age, and up to 25% in those 85 years of age and older.

Delirium

Delirium is an acute change in mental functioning that can be accompanied by symptoms of restlessness, incoherence of speech and thought, illusions, and hallucinations. It can present over a few hours or days, and may fluctuate over the course of the same day. It has been referred to as "an acute state of confusion" and can be reversible in many cases.

The estimated prevalence of delirium in the population older than 65 years of age is 1% to 2%. As age increases, so does prevalence, and delirium is greatest among elderly residents of long-term care facilities. Prevalence in the general public older than 85 years of age is approximately 10% to 14%.

Delirium is frequently seen in elderly patients who are hospitalized. It has been identified in 40% of patients hospitalized in ICUs. Emergency department staff might expect to see 10% to 30% of patients with delirium, as it has a sudden onset and is frightening to the patient and the family.

Delirium can be a result of substance use and substance withdrawal. It can also result from a medical condition such as liver failure or as a reaction to a combination of medications.

Neurodegenerative Disorders

Neurodegenerative disorders are often synonymous with neurocognitive disease, as many patients have neurocognitive decline as part of their presentation. These disorders characteristically produce a loss of neuronal structural integrity, and some also cause increased accumulation of protein in the brain. The most common neurodegenerative diseases are Alzheimer's disease, Parkinson's disease, and multiple sclerosis (see Figures 10.2 through 10.4). Alzheimer's disease, unlike Parkinson's disease and multiple sclerosis, is more common among the elderly. All three cause cognitive decline, and currently there is no cure for any of them. This chapter focuses on Alzheimer's disease. Multiple sclerosis is discussed in detail in Chapter 13.

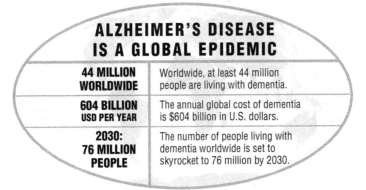

Figure 10.2 Prevalence of Alzheimer's disease. *Source: Adapted from Townsend (2015).*

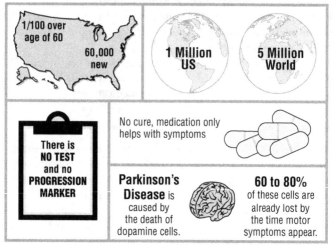

Figure 10.3 Prevalence of Parkinson's disease. *Source: Adapted from Michael J. Fox Foundation for Parkinson's Research (n.d.).*

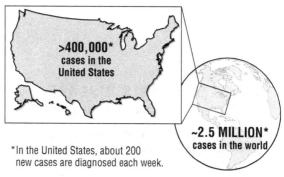

Figure 10.4 Prevalence of multiple sclerosis. *Source: Adapted from Pietrangelo and Higuera (2015).*

Fast Facts in the Spotlight

Neurodegenerative disorders that cause neurocognitive impairment are not limited to the elderly. Although some of these disorders, such as Alzheimer's disease, Lewy body disease, frontotemporal lobar degeneration, and vascular disease are more prevalent in older adults, others, such as traumatic brain injury, prion disease, HIV infection, Parkinson's disease, and substance- or medication-related degenerative disorder affect people of all ages. All of these disorders cause impairment in one or more cognitive domains and have a significant impact on the patients' and family members' lives.

OVERVIEW OF NEUROCOGNITIVE AND NEURODEGENERATIVE DISORDERS

The signature symptom of a neurocognitive disorder is alteration in thoughts, memory, and information processing. Patients with many of the neurodegenerative disorders also have symptoms of neurocognitive decline, which is why these disorders are discussed in this chapter.

Diagnosis of a neurocognitive disorder is made when a patient demonstrates an acquired decline in cognition involving one or more cognitive domains. The four domains of cognitive functioning are:

1. Recent memory
2. Language
3. Visuospatial ability
4. Executive function

These cognitive deficits can impair a person's ability for independent living, and can be caused by a neurodegenerative disorder as well as some other mental illnesses.

MAJOR VERSUS MILD NEUROCOGNITIVE DISORDERS

Major neurocognitive disorders are disorders in which the decline in cognitive functioning related to executive functioning, memory, attention, language, social cognition, or perceptual and motor skills is grave enough to significantly impact the patient's activities of daily living. *Mild neurocognitive disorders* are those in which the decline from previous functioning is modest and the patient's activities of daily living are not significantly affected.

As earlier chapters have emphasized, many psychiatric disorders, such as major depression (see Chapter 6) and schizophrenia (see Chapter 5), can affect cognitive functioning. Therefore, the patient who presents with decline in cognitive deficits should be evaluated to rule out the presence of another mental illness.

RECOGNIZING SIGNS AND SYMPTOMS OF NEUROCOGNITIVE AND NEURODEGENERATIVE DISORDERS

The signature sign of a neurocognitive disorder is alteration in the ability to process, store, and act upon information. This decline in cognitive functioning is not due to another psychiatric condition. As with the other disorders, the impairments in cognition and function are multidimensional, occurring on a spectrum from mild to severe. Patients are referred to as low or high functioning, depending on their ability to perform independent activities of daily living. Patients are evaluated using specific neuropsychological tests that can compare an individual's level of functioning with that of a person of the same age, level of education, and culture without neurocognitive decline. Common symptoms and signs noted in patients with impaired cognitive function include:

- Changes in ability to store recent memories
- Increased agitation and irritability
- Confusion
- Depression (may or may not be present)

Evaluating Presenting Symptoms

Delirium

Delirium is an acute medical emergency. Patients experiencing delirium have an increased hospital mortality rate that is 2 to 20 times the rate of other patients.

Symptoms usually develop quickly, within hours or days, and can include hyperactivity, agitation, and psychotic symptoms such as hallucinations (auditory, visual, or sensory). Psychomotor agitation is usually present, and patients may manifest increased wandering, pacing, and often verbal outbursts. Family members may report that the patient is collecting and hoarding items at home; engaging in repetitive, purposeless behaviors; and acting outside of his or her normal behaviors.

Alzheimer's Disease and Other Neurodegenerative Disorders

The patient with a neurocognitive disorder will demonstrate certain indicators on initial assessment. There may be an indication of poor judgment or an inability to make decisions. When administered the mini-mental state exam, the patient may be unable to demonstrate recent memory skills or know the date or season. The patient or a family member may report an inability to keep track of personal items, remember where the car is parked, or recall where items should be placed in the refrigerator. It is not unusual to find that the patient is also experiencing depression along with the cognitive decline.

The Alzheimer's Association (2017) provides a list of the early signs and symptoms of the disease, which can be presented to the family as a referral if they are interested in learning more. They include:

- Memory loss
- Problem-solving challenges
- Inability to complete once-familiar tasks
- Confusion related to time or place
- Difficulty with visual images and spatial relationships
- Problems retrieving or remembering words when speaking or writing
- Misplacing things and being unable to "retrace" the steps to find them
- Demonstrating a decrease in judgment, or showing poor judgment
- Social isolation
- Mood and personality changes

MEDICATIONS USED TO TREAT NEUROCOGNITIVE AND NEURODEGENERATIVE DISORDERS

As this chapter has indicated, many different disease entities can result in neurocognitive decline. Interventions and medications must be tailored to the cause, symptoms, and definitive diagnosis.

Delirium

Because the causes of delirium are so diverse, treatment includes keeping the patient safe and determining the etiology of his or her symptoms. It is particularly important to identify any rapidly correctable causative factor (e.g., medication reaction or infection). The airway must be protected, and the patient carefully monitored.

A neuroleptic (antipsychotic, second-generation) medication such as risperidone, olanzapine, or quetiapine is sometimes used to relieve some of the symptoms of delirium. Mundigler et al. (2002) reported on the use of melatonin in treating patients with delirium, as altered levels of melatonin had previously been identified in these patients. Lorazepam (Ativan) is a short-acting benzodiazepine that can be given intramuscularly or intravenously for sedation and is also effective when delirium is associated with withdrawal from another drug. The patient should be closely monitored for any changes in level of consciousness, and the airway maintained and stabilized, during treatment.

Alzheimer's Disease

Generally, when a patient demonstrates a decline in cognition that is related to a neurocognitive disorder, one or more of the following medications are considered for treatment.

For Mild to Moderate Alzheimer's Disease

- Cholinesterase inhibitors, including donepezil (Aricept), galantamine (Razadyne), and rivastigmine (Exelon)
- These drugs can be expensive, and side effects include insomnia, nausea, muscle cramps, diarrhea, and reduced appetite

For Moderate to Severe Alzheimer's Disease

- Memantine (Namenda)—an N-methyl-D-aspartate (NMDA) antagonist—may delay the progression of symptoms of cognitive decline through glutamate regulation
- Donepezil (Aricept, Namzaric)
- Antidepressants
  - Selective serotonin reuptake inhibitors, including sertraline, citalopram, escitalopram, and paroxetine (see Chapter 7)
  - Trazodone
- Anticonvulsants (mood stabilizers) (see Chapter 6)
  - Sodium valproate
  - Carbamazepine

THERAPEUTIC AND ENVIRONMENTAL STRATEGIES USED TO TREAT THESE DISORDERS

Nonpharmacological interventions in neurodegenerative disorders are focused on slowing the progression of impairment in activities of daily life. Neurodegenerative diseases are both diverse in their presentation and complex in their functional impact on the patient's biological system. Through maximizing a person's ability to carry out daily functions and slow the loss of self-care independence, the quality of life can be improved. The following interventions have been demonstrated to provide moderate positive effects on quality of life.

- *Occupational therapy* involving encouraging and facilitating the patient in exercising activities and skills required in everyday functioning
- *Environmental/milieu therapy* through structured environments that provide programs; examples include:
  - Day program or continual care/extended care
  - Behavior modification program
- *Family education* for safety issues and de-escalation
- *Referral* for community and caregiver support

Table 10.1

Nursing Diagnosis and ICD-10 Nomenclature for Neurocognitive and Neurodegenerative Disorders

Nursing diagnoses	ICD-10 codes
Self-care deficit	The ICD-10 codes relate to the level of cognitive impairment and neurodegenerative disease; a few of those related to delirium and Alzheimer's disease include:
Ineffective self-health management	
Risk for imbalanced nutrition	
Chronic confusion	
Risk-prone behavior	Unspecified delirium (R41.0)
Risk for self-directed or other-directed violence	Delirium due to known physiological condition (F05)
Caregiver role strain	Alzheimer's disease (G30.9)
	Mild cognitive impairment (G31.84)

Sources: Herdman & NANDA (2012); ICD10Data.com (n.d.).

MATCHING NURSING DIAGNOSIS AND MEDICAL DIAGNOSIS

Table 10.1 correlates nursing diagnoses with the ICD-10 codes for neurocognitive and neurodegenerative disorders.

SPOTLIGHT ON THE UNIT: DELIRIUM IN THE MEDI-CLINIC

It is a cold winter afternoon in an urban medi-clinic. Nurse X immediately notices an older White woman who appears to be in her 60s. It is snowing outside and most patients in the waiting room are still wearing their outer coats, but this woman is dressed in shorts. She is pacing in circles while yelling periodically at no one in particular.

A teenage boy rushes through the clinic door yelling, "Grandma, Grandma! What happened? What are you doing? Grandpa's on his way. It's going to be ok. . . ." The woman stops, stares at him for a moment, then resumes her pacing, more agitated than before. "Go away . . . go away . . . go away," she repeats to no one.

The boy goes to the front desk and tells the receptionist, "My name is Danny Rone. That's my grandma. A few hours ago she started acting crazy and now she is really scaring me. I don't know what's happening to her. This isn't like her at all! Can someone please help her?"

Within minutes, an older man comes into the clinic, and calls out "Daria!" to the woman, who again stops her pacing and stares at him. "What is happening to me?" she cries out. As the older man joins the boy at the front desk, he tells the receptionist, "She didn't feel well this morning. She had a cold and a urinary tract infection, and she took some medications when she got up that the doctor prescribed. Then, a few hours ago she really started to act crazy. Please help us!"

- What might the problem be?
- What questions do you need to ask the family?
- How can you help Daria?

Further Reading

De Lange, E., Vergaak, P. F., & van der Meer, K. (2013). Prevalence, presentation and prognosis of delirium in older people in the population, at home and in long term care: A review. *International Journal of Geriatric Psychiatry*, 28(2), 127–134.

Foster, E. R. (2014). Themes from the special issue on neurodegenerative diseases: What have we learned, and where can we go from here? *American Journal of Occupational Therapy*, 68(1), 6–8. doi:10.5014/ajot.2014.009910

National Institute on Aging. (2016). Alzheimer's disease education and referral center. Retrieved from https://www.nia.nih.gov/alzheimers/publication/alzheimers-disease-medications-fact-sheet

Townsend, M. (2015). *Psychiatric nursing: Assessment, care plans, and medications*. Philadelphia, PA: F. A. Davis.

References

Alzheimer's Association. (2017). 10 early signs and symptoms of Alzheimer's. Retrieved from http://www.alz.org/alzheimers_disease_10_signs_of_alzheimers.asp

Herdman, T. H., & North American Nursing Diagnosis Association. (2012). *Nursing diagnoses: Definitions & classification 2012–2014*. Chichester, United Kingdom: Wiley-Blackwell.

ICD10Data.com. (n.d.). Retrieved from http://www.icd10data.com

Lobo, A., Launer, L. J., Fratiglioni, L., Andersen, K., DiCarlo, A., Breteler, M. M., . . . & Hofman, A. (2000). Prevalence of dementia and major subtypes in Europe: A collaborative study of population-based cohorts. Neurologic diseases in the elderly research group. *Neurology*, 54(11 suppl. 5): S4–S9.

Michael J. Fox Foundation for Parkinson's Research. (n.d.). What is Parkinson's? Retrieved from https://www.michaeljfox.org/page.html?what-is-parkinsons-infographic

Mundigler, G., Delle-Karth, G., Koreny, M., Zehetgruber, M., Steindl-Munda, P., Marktl, W., . . . Siostrzonek, P. (2002). Impaired circadian rhythm of melatonin secretion in sedated critically ill patients with severe sepsis. *Critical Care Medicine*, 30, 536–540.

Pietrangelo, A., & Higuera, V. (2015). Multiple sclerosis by the numbers: Facts, statistics, and you. Retrieved from http://www.healthline.com/health/multiple-sclerosis/facts-statistics-infographic

Townsend, T. (2015). Never forget—we can't stop Alzheimer's (yet) but we can preserve memories! [Blog post]. Retrieved from http://weeva.com/blog/2015/12/18/never-forget-we-cant-stop-alzheimers-yet-but-we-can-preserve-memories

van der Flier, W. M., & Scheltens, P. (2005). Epidemiology and risk factors of dementia. *Journal of Neurology, Neurosurgery & Psychiatry*, 76(Suppl. 5). Retrieved from http://jnnp.bmj.com/content/76/suppl_5/v2

III

Medical Diagnosis and Mental Illness: Symptom Sharing

11

Medical Diagnosis and Symptom Sharing: Metabolic Disease

In this chapter, you will learn:

- What we mean by confounding symptoms, and why knowing about them is important to nurses
- Common symptoms that may be noted in patients with specific metabolic diseases who do not have a psychiatric diagnosis
- Metabolic symptoms (acquired and hereditary) in presenting patients that can be mistaken for psychiatric symptoms
- Nursing actions to address patients' confounding symptoms

The three chapters that constitute Part III identify psychiatric symptoms that are most commonly shared with metabolic (Chapter 11), respiratory (Chapter 12), and neurological (Chapter 13) diseases, and briefly discuss the perils of not investigating for other causes when patients present with these symptoms. Each chapter provides an overview of specific, more common diseases, highlighting the shared psychiatric symptoms as well as the other accompanying signs of disease.

Specific questions that can be asked of the patient to help identify the causes of his or her symptoms are included. These are not intended to be comprehensive, but offer a starting point from which the nurse can gather more information about the patient. Finally, each chapter describes how the registered nurse (RN) and the advanced practice registered nurse (APRN) can intervene when managing a patient with shared symptoms of psychiatric disease. Even though the patient has a metabolic, respiratory, or neurological condition, he or she may also be experiencing a co-occurring psychiatric problem. It is our job to get all the facts before beginning any treatment.

Fast Facts in the Spotlight

When evaluating the diagnostic criteria for psychiatric diseases, one of the stipulations is that the symptoms are not caused by, or attributable to, an existing or possible medical condition. This caveat is important, because treatment of the symptom in a patient with a medical condition may be very different from that for a patient with a psychiatric disorder, and mistreatment could do harm to the patient.

Identifying the cause of the patient's symptoms may require a more thorough examination of the facts. Many somatic and psychological symptoms originate from different metabolic diseases. Figuring out how to help your patient may place you in the role of a detective of sorts, following the clues to solve a mystery. The "clues" in this chapter are presenting symptoms that are commonly believed to be of psychiatric origin but might well have a basis in a metabolic disease.

CONFOUNDING SYMPTOMS

The word *confound* means to confuse, or to mistakenly treat one thing as another. In this context, *confounding symptoms* are symptoms that are shared by different disorders, which increases the likelihood of mistaking one disease for another. We could simply say *shared symptoms*, as they are shared; however, trying to establish a possible diagnosis on the basis of symptoms alone, without investigating past medical history, current medications, blood work, and results of other medical tests, can lead to incorrect treatments and less than optimum outcomes.

Specific observations we make during the initial assessment include the patient's state of consciousness; orientation to time, place, and person; personal hygiene; ability to concentrate and pay attention to the questions being asked; mood or affect; and clarity of thought as demonstrated by speech. Each of these assessments provides a window into the patient's psychological functioning, but it may also be the first indication of other disorders that are metabolic in nature. Follow-up questions, information from family members when available, and examination of the patient's history of hospitalization, sleep hygiene, and family history will help to clear the haze of the mystery.

Excellent nursing care requires engaging in the nursing process and assessing the patient. Your assessment of the patient presenting with psychological symptoms should alert you to start a thorough investigation into the facts!

SHARED SYMPTOMS

The following symptoms are shared by both metabolic and psychiatric disorders:

- Fatigue
- Depression
- Slowed mental processes
- Weight gain
- Decreased concentration
- Personality changes
- Anxiety
- Dull expressions
- Social withdrawal

Fast Facts in the Spotlight

Sometimes patients with dysthymia or depression, or both, will be placed on levothyroxine (Synthroid) as a primary or adjunctive medication to improve the symptoms of depression, without the patient having the clinical diagnosis of hypothyroidism.

COMMON METABOLIC DISEASES WITH POSSIBLE PSYCHIATRIC SYMPTOMS

Hypothyroidism

Hypothyroidism (low levels of thyroid hormone) is more commonly diagnosed in women, and prevalence increases with age. Patients with hypothyroidism who are misdiagnosed with depression may be further misdiagnosed as being treatment resistant, since the use of antidepressants will not correct their underlying thyroid problem.

Hypothyroidism can be caused by radiation to the neck, insufficient iodine in the diet, and thyroid cancer. In Hashimoto's thyroiditis, an autoimmune disease, the presence of circulating antibodies interferes with iodine uptake. Often symptoms first appear during pregnancy. Some medications (e.g., lithium) can also cause hypothyroidism.

Presenting Psychiatric Symptoms

Fatigue, depression, slowed mental processes, weight gain, decreased concentration, personality changes, dull expression, deep/hoarse voice, constipation, and intolerance to heat and cold

Other Symptoms

Psychosis reaction and delirium with hallucinations, agitation, and disorientation; may be referred to as *myxedema madness* (rare, but can occur)

Questions to Ask

- How long have you been feeling this way?
- Do you know if anyone in your family takes Synthroid, or has been diagnosed with thyroid disease?
- Have you ever taken lithium?
- Have you had radiation to your neck area?
- Have you ever been told that you, or a family member, has a "slow thyroid"?
- Are you pregnant?
- Do you know of any history of mental illness in your family? (Provide a menu: depression, alcoholism, etc.)

Interventions

- *RN*: Interview, observe, chart, and report. Share your observations with your team and the treating/prescribing health care professional.
- *APRN*: Same as RN plus lab tests—thyroid-stimulating hormone (TSH), thyroxine (T_4), triiodothyronine (T_3), and free T_4.

Hyperthyroidism

As with hypothyroidism, hyperthyroidism (high levels of thyroid hormone) is more commonly diagnosed in women, and similarly, prevalence increases with age. Graves' disease, an autoimmune disorder, accounts for most cases of hyperactive thyroid disease.

Hyperthyroidism can be caused by radioactive iodine treatment, and by thyroid medication noncompliance. Postpartum diagnosis of hyperthyroidism is not unusual. As with hypothyroidism, taking lithium can be a factor in the development of hyperthyroidism.

Presenting Psychiatric Symptoms

Hyperactivity, anxiety, insomnia, concentration deficit, depression, and emotional lability

Other Symptoms

Palpitations, muscle weakness, tachycardia, weight loss, increased bowel movements, menstrual irregularity, difficulty getting pregnant, psychosis, fatigue, apathy, and agitation (older adults)

Questions to Ask

- How long have you been feeling this way?
- Do you know if anyone in your family has been diagnosed with thyroid disease?
- Have you ever taken lithium?
- Are you pregnant, or have you recently had a child?
- Do you know of any history of mental illness in your family? (Provide a menu: depression, alcoholism, etc.)

Interventions

- *RN*: Assess, chart, and report. Share your observations with your team and the treating/prescribing health care professional.
- *APRN*: Same as RN plus lab test for TSH, radioiodine uptake test, and thyroid scan.

Acromegaly

Acromegaly is usually caused by a benign tumor of the pituitary gland and less commonly by tumors of the hypothalamus that result in production of excessive growth hormone. This is a rare syndrome, with onset usually around 40 to 50 years of age.

Presenting Psychiatric Symptoms

Fatigue, headaches, impotence, depression, irritability, impairment of recent memory, lack of sex drive, sleep disturbance secondary to sleep apnea, fluctuation of mood, and social withdrawal

Other Symptoms

Excessive bleeding or irregularities in menstruation, acne, organ enlargement, and nonpregnancy-related lactation

Questions to Ask

- Has anyone in your family been diagnosed with acromegaly?
- Do you know of any history of mental illness in your family? (Provide a menu: depression, alcoholism, etc.)

Interventions

- *RN*: Identify whether there has been a recent growth spurt, or changes in shoe or hand size. Assess history; document and share information.
- *APRN*: Same as RN plus lab tests—insulin-like growth factor 1 (IGF-1), oral glucose tolerance test (OGTT); imaging tests.

Cushing's Syndrome

Cushing's syndrome is usually caused by prolonged use of corticosteroid medications, resulting in hypercortisolism. Tumors of the adrenal glands or other adrenocorticotropic hormone (ACTH)–producing glands can also result in Cushing's syndrome.

Presenting Psychiatric Symptoms

Insomnia, mania, depression, emotional lability, cognitive disturbances, and confusion

Other Symptoms

Round, ruddy face; hypertension; fat pads on upper back and collar bone; decreased muscle in the extremities; and truncal obesity

Questions to Ask

- Have you been taking corticosteroids for a long time? (Provide a menu.)
- What medications do you normally take? Have you stopped taking any of them recently?
- Do you know if anyone in your family has been treated for a psychiatric disorder (e.g., depression, anxiety, alcoholism)?

Interventions

- *RN*: Assess mental function, environmental awareness, and mood. Observe for skin breakdown as these patients are slow to heal. Document findings and share with your team.
- *APRN*: Same as RN plus overnight dexamethasone suppression test; 24-hour urinary free cortisol level; and computed tomography (CT) or magnetic resonance imaging (MRI) scan of adrenals, if indicated.

Diabetes Mellitus

Diabetes mellitus (DM) is a disorder that results from insufficient pancreatic production of insulin. DM and depression have been identified as having a "bidirectional association—both influencing each other in multiple ways" (Balhara, 2011). In other words, depression is a risk factor for developing diabetes and vice versa. Patients with diabetes mellitus are at higher risk for depression than people without DM. The rate of major depressive disorder in people diagnosed with DM is between 8% and 18% (average of 12%), and for milder forms of depression between 15% and 35% (Andreoulakis, Hyphantis, Kandylis, & Iacovides, 2012). This comorbidity significantly impacts patient outcomes. Patients with co-occurring diabetes and depression are less likely to adhere to their medications and have a poorer quality of life. The prevalence of DM in people older than 65 years of age is 12%.

Presenting Psychiatric Symptoms

Depression, cognitive impairment, fatigue, and blurred vision

Other Symptoms

Hyperglycemia; polyuria; polydipsia; dry mouth; dry, itchy skin; slow-healing cuts; unplanned weight loss; nausea and vomiting; and pain and numbness in feet or legs, or both

Questions to Ask

- Have you been diagnosed with sugar in the blood, high blood sugar, or diabetes?
- Does anyone in your family have diabetes?
- Have you been more thirsty than usual lately?
- Do you find that you have to urinate more frequently recently?

- Do you take any "sugar" medications, like insulin or Glucotrol?
- Has anyone in your family been treated for, or diagnosed with, a psychiatric disorder?

Interventions

- *RN*: Identify any risks for infections; assess mental status and physical status. Document all findings and share with the health care team.
- *APRN*: Same as RN plus test blood glucose, serum osmolality, hemoglobin/hematocrit (Hb/Hct), and blood urea nitrogen/creatinine (BUN/Cr).

Acute Porphyrias

Porphyria is an inherited disease that leads to deficiency in the ability to make heme in the hemoglobin due to a buildup of porphyrin in the blood. Rarely seen in prepubescent and postmenopausal patients, this blood condition interferes with the ability of hemoglobin to bind to iron and carry oxygen. Patients may die during an untreated episode from respiratory arrest secondary to paralysis of lung muscles.

Presenting Psychiatric Symptoms

Depression, apathy, catatonia, anxiety, restlessness, confusion, disorientation, paranoia, with complaints of numbness, tingling, and weakness in the muscles. The symptoms appear intermittently, and the patient can return to baseline functioning between episodes.

Other Symptoms

Acute pain, nausea, vomiting, high blood pressure, headache, and seizures

Questions to Ask

- Have you or any other family member experienced these kinds of episodes or been diagnosed with porphyria variegate?
- Have you been drinking alcohol or taking drugs recently? (Can precipitate an episode.)
- Do you frequently have episodes of abdominal pain?
- Do you know of any history of mental illness in your family? (Provide a menu: depression, alcoholism, etc.)

Interventions

- *RN*: Patient education—alcohol and drugs can precipitate an episode. A diet high in carbohydrates could reduce frequency of attacks. Birth control pills have assisted in hormonal control.
- *APRN*: Same as RN plus test to identify molecules indicating impaired metabolism. Check for urine that darkens when left in the light.

TAKE-AWAY

With current statistics showing that one in four Americans have a mental disorder, the need for every nurse to engage in mental health nursing is imperative. Likewise, because many nonpsychiatric disorders share symptoms with psychiatric disorders, it is important that the source of a patient's "confounding" symptoms be adequately investigated.

Further Reading

Bonnot, O., Herrera, P. M., Tordjman, S., & Walterfang, M. (2015). Secondary psychosis induced by metabolic disorders. *Frontiers in Neuroscience*, *9*, 177. doi:10.3389/fnins.2015.00177

Demily, C., & Sedel, F. (2014). Psychiatric manifestations of treatable hereditary metabolic disorders in adults. *Annals of General Psychiatry*, *13*, 27. doi:10.1186/s12991-014-0027-x

Nouwen, A., Winkley, K., Twisk, J., Lloyd, C. E., Peyrot, M., Ismail, K., & Pouwer, F. (2010). Type 2 diabetes mellitus as a risk factor for the onset of depression: A systematic review and meta-analysis. *Diabetologia*, *53*(12), 2480–2486.

Schildkrout, B. (2014). *Masquerading Symptoms*. Hoboken, NJ: Wiley.

References

Andreoulakis, E., Hyphantis, T., Kandylis, D., & Iacovides, A. (2012). Depression in diabetes mellitus: A comprehensive review. *Hippokratia*, *16*(3), 205–214.

Balhara, Y. P. S. (2011). Diabetes and psychiatric disorders. *Indian Journal of Endocrinology and Metabolism*, *15*(4), 274–283. doi:10.4103/2230-8210.85579

Website Resources

American Thyroid Association: www.thyroid.org/thyroid-function-tests

Mayo Clinic: www.mayoclinic.org/diseases-conditions/acromegaly/diagnosis-treatment/diagnosis/dxc-20177632

Mayo Clinic: www.mayoclinic.org/diseases-conditions/hyperthyroidism/basics/definition/con-20020986

NurseLabs: www.nurselabs.com/cushing-syndrome-nursing-management

12

Medical Diagnosis and Symptom Sharing: Respiratory Disease

In this chapter, you will learn:

- Symptoms that are shared by psychiatric disorders and respiratory diseases
- Common symptoms that may be noted in patients with specific respiratory diseases who do not have a psychiatric diagnosis
- Respiratory disorders (acquired and hereditary) in presenting patients that can be mistaken for psychiatric signs and symptoms
- Nursing actions to address patients' confounding symptoms

CONFOUNDING SYMPTOMS

Breathing is central to life. Just try holding your breath for a few seconds and appreciate how it affects your heart rate, your thoughts, and, of course, your comfort. Now consider how you would react if the ability to take the next breath was not within your power to control. Loss of the ability to breathe is a real and immediate danger to life, and as such can precipitate any number of anxiety reactions, including panic attacks. Understanding a patient's history and having the strategies necessary to reduce both the anxiety of the physical discomfort of respiratory distress and the fear many people have when coming for medical treatment is a nursing imperative. As the health care professionals who usually are the first to sit with patients, and who will spend the most therapeutic time with them, nurses have the chance to help patients feel less frightened and more comfortable with the upcoming treatments they will be receiving. Unfortunately, perceived lack of caring or attention from the nursing staff can have a negative impact on a patient's well-being.

Fast Facts in the Spotlight

When we do not approach our patients with empathy and an open mind we can, especially with those experiencing a respiratory disorder, exacerbate the illness. Consider the following patient response: "It felt like I simply could not breathe in. I was looking at the nurses and the doctors, but I could not speak and I was hanging on the doorway and trying to control my panic. I thought that the staff were not taking it seriously and it was making me panic" (Browningrigg, 2007).

Of course, just as with metabolic diseases, specific observations we make during the initial assessment will help guide our interventions. The initial assessment should include observation of skin color, use of accessory muscles for breathing, level of consciousness, level of attention, mood, and clarity of thought. If the patient is older, or has a history of smoking and alcohol use, it is important to reserve any opinion you might have about the cause of the respiratory distress or clarity of thinking until all the facts are collected. A long-standing respiratory condition can affect mental processing, mood, and ability to concentrate. Providing oxygen to a patient with a history of lung disease, whose body has adjusted to lower oxygen levels, can cause harm rather than support. Each person whom we treat has his or her own story and history and needs to be examined in the same way we would approach a new baby.

Impact of Chronic Lung Diseases on Emotional Well-Being

People living with a respiratory illness, from the common cold to terminal lung cancer, experience psychological distress. The more acute the onset and the more chronic the experience of respiratory failure, the more intense will be the psychological symptoms. Not being able to catch your breath affects every aspect of daily living. Acute as well as chronic experiences of dyspnea can cause stress, anxiety, fear of death, panic, irritability, and often outright anger. Reduced oxygen intake to the lungs decreases available oxygen to the brain, which can result in memory loss, confusion, and stroke. The presence of these symptoms may identify a co-occurring psychological disorder; however, sometimes these signal a real and present danger of respiratory failure that needs to be attended to immediately.

SHARED SYMPTOMS

The following symptoms are shared by both respiratory and psychiatric disorders:

- Fatigue
- Restlessness
- Agitation
- Decreased mental acuity
- Difficulty concentrating
- Confusion and disorientation
- Seizures
- Alteration in consciousness
- Hallucinations
- Delirium

COMMON RESPIRATORY DISEASES WITH POSSIBLE PSYCHIATRIC SYMPTOMS

Carbon Monoxide Poisoning

Carbon monoxide poisoning occurs as a result of exposure to high levels of carbon monoxide (CO). Exposure may be acute or chronic, with low sub-lethal level contact. Patients may not be aware of their exposure to CO, as it is found in car exhaust, solvents, and in the exhaust of some nonelectric generators. CO poisoning is the second most common cause of nonmedicinal poisoning death in the United States (Sircar et al., 2015). See Figure 12.1.

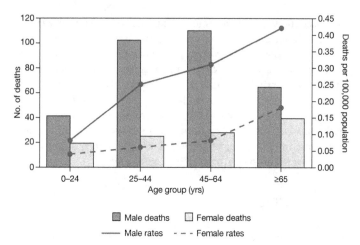

Figure 12.1 Average annual number of deaths and death rates from unintentional, non–fire-related carbon monoxide poisoning by sex and age group. *Source: Centers for Disease Control and Prevention (2014).*

Presenting Psychiatric Symptoms

Fatigue, restlessness, agitation, decreased mental acuity, difficulty concentrating, confusion and disorientation, alteration in consciousness, seizures, hallucinations, and delirium. Later symptoms include echolalia, mutism, ataxia, and bizarre behaviors.

Other Symptoms

Generic flu symptoms, dizziness, shortness of breath, complaints of chronic fatigue, chest pain, diarrhea and vomiting, muscle aches and pains, tachycardia, and nausea. Symptoms can be delayed, occurring 2 to 40 days after exposure (Tomaszewski, 2015).

Questions to Ask

- How long have you been feeling this way?
- Is anyone with whom you work or live experiencing the same kinds of symptoms?
- Do you routinely work with paint strippers or solvents?
- Do you have a wood-burning stove in your home?
- Do you have a CO detector in your home or workplace?
- Do you have a nonelectric generator in your home?

- Have you been scuba diving? (A faulty diving air compressor can cause CO poisoning.)
- Have you tried to commit suicide?
- Do you know of any history of mental illness in your family? (Provide a menu: depression, alcoholism, etc.)

Interventions

- *RN*: Interview, observe, chart, and report. Beware—the pulse oximeter may give you a normal, but incorrect, reading. Share your observations with your team and the treating/prescribing health care professional immediately as this can be a life-threatening situation. Be prepared to do CPR.
- *APRN*: Same as RN plus administer 100% oxygen.

Hypoxia and Altitude Sickness

Hypoxia occurs when the lungs are unable to take in a sufficient supply of oxygen to supply to the brain. Although the brain makes up only 2% of our total body weight, it needs 25% of the oxygen we inhale! Hypoxia is often associated with other long-standing, chronic lung disorders such as emphysema, chronic obstructive pulmonary disease (COPD), asthma, and lung cancer. As such, hypoxia itself can be an outcome of any medical issue that would result in decreased oxygenation, including pneumonia, heart failure, and sleep apnea. People with sleep apnea may not be aware of their lack of oxygen during sleep, and the possibility of hypoxia may surprise them.

Fast Facts in the Spotlight

Patients with chronic lung diseases probably have physically accommodated to their reduced oxygen levels and may be especially susceptible to rapid deterioration as a result of lack of oxygen to the brain. Also remember that the body that has acclimated and adjusted to lower oxygen and higher CO levels may be adversely affected by too much oxygen!

Presenting Psychiatric Symptoms

Depression, disorientation, possible euphoria, short-term memory loss, uncooperative behavior, cognitive changes, confusion, and anxiety

Other Symptoms

Dyspnea, seizures, impaired motor coordination, altered state of consciousness, visual agnosias, use of accessory muscles when breathing, and confabulation secondary to memory loss

Questions to Ask

- Do you have a history of respiratory illness?
- Have you recently had the flu, congestion, or pneumonia?
- Do you have a history of cardiac problems?
- Did this breathing difficulty happen suddenly?
- Were you with anyone else who can say what happened?
- Do you smoke (cigarettes, e-cigs, marijuana, other)?
- Have you taken any drugs that might make you sleepy?
- Do you work with chemicals?
- Do you have a CO monitor where you live or work?
- Have you ever been told you have sleep apnea?
- Do you use a C-PAP machine at night?

Interventions

- *RN*: Assess, chart, and report. Share your observations with your team and the treating/prescribing health care professional. It is especially important to collect a good history. Monitor vital signs and level of consciousness closely.
- *APRN*: Same as RN plus determine the safe level of oxygen for this patient, with careful consideration of any long-standing pulmonary problems.

Sleep Apnea

Sleep apnea has been mentioned in the preceding Hypoxia section; however, many people who have this condition may not be aware of it until one or more psychiatric symptoms cause them or a loved one to become concerned. Sleep apnea, or the lack of respirations during sleep, can last from a few seconds to a number of minutes. The person may awaken during sleep due to the snoring or loud choking sound that occurs when breathing restarts.

Obstructive sleep apnea has a mechanical etiology and is often caused by obesity, enlarged tonsils, or other tracheal partial obstructions. People with obstructive sleep apnea usually snore.

Central sleep apnea, on the other hand, is due to mixed brain signals, which do not trigger the respiratory muscles to move. This is not a common diagnosis and may occur with or without obstructive sleep apnea. Central sleep apnea, when not combined with obstructive sleep apnea, does not include snoring.

Sleep apnea is a serious condition that can lead to hypertension, heart attack, and heart failure. In women, there is an associated increased risk of heart failure.

Presenting Psychiatric Symptoms

Chronic fatigue and exhaustion in the absence of strenuous activity; insomnia, hypersomnia, inattention, irritability, and moodiness

Other Symptoms

Chronic dry mouth on awaking, sore throat, and morning headaches

Questions to Ask

Use the STOP BANG questionnaire (body mass index, age, neck size, and gender), as well as the following questions:

- Have you been waking up with a headache?
- Do you wake up at night, sometimes choking?
- Have people said that you snore?
- Can your snoring be heard through closed doors?
- Have you ever been diagnosed with a sleep disorder?
- Is your BMI over 35?
- Is your neck circumference greater than 40?

Interventions

- *RN*: Assess, chart, and report. Share your observations with your team and the treating/prescribing health care professional. Use questionnaires as needed (e.g., the STOP BANG questionnaire; see references for website resources).
- *APRN*: Same as RN plus evaluation for continuous positive airway pressure (CPAP).

Chronic Obstructive Pulmonary Disease

Asthma

Asthma is a chronic respiratory disease that obstructs airway flow due to spasms in the bronchi. The inflammation causes a narrowing of the airways, making breathing difficult. It is one of the most common

U.S. chronic health disorders (Kewalramani, Bollinger, & Postolache, 2008). A relationship has been identified between mood disorders and asthma, and patients who have asthma were found to be twice as likely to have a mood disorder as patients without asthma (Lieshout & MacQueen, 2012).

Presenting Psychiatric Symptoms
Anxiety, panic, fear, and depression

Other Symptoms
Shortness of breath, chest tightness, and air hunger

Questions to Ask
- Do you have a history of allergies?
- Have you ever had an asthma attack?
- Do you have trouble breathing when you are doing simple tasks, or in the fall or spring?

Interventions
- *RN*: Assess, chart, and report. Listen to lung sounds. Share your observations with your team and the treating/prescribing health care professional.
- *APRN*: Same as RN plus full physical exam, including spirometry and lung function tests.
- Referral to a pulmonary specialist.

Chronic Bronchitis and Emphysema

Patients with chronic bronchitis and emphysema present with similar signs and symptoms, and both diseases reduce the available oxygen to the brain. Both are considered chronic obstructive pulmonary diseases. The most common causes are smoking and air pollution. Bronchitis is an inflammation of the bronchi, causing infection and irritation of the lung's air passages. Emphysema, on the other hand, is a disease that destroys the alveoli, resulting in chronic shortness of breath and air hunger.

Psychiatric Symptoms
Panic, anxiety, fear, phobias, and cognitive changes

Other Symptoms
Coughing, wheezing, and chronic exhaustion

Questions to Ask
- Have you ever been told you have a breathing illness?

- Are there any specific events or activities that make breathing harder?
- Do you take any medicines (prescribed or over the counter) to help you breathe better?

Interventions

- Provide relief of breathing difficulties (elevate the head of the bed, provide extra pillows, and give as-needed nasal cannula oxygen when ordered).
- Keep call bell and other items within easy reach of the patient to reduce the anxiety associated with calling for help when needed.
- Prevent complications: Monitor antibiotic therapy for bacterial infections, evaluate the patient's nutritional needs, and investigate availability of pulmonary rehabilitation.

TAKE-AWAY

We have reviewed some of the more common respiratory diseases that often develop or coexist with psychiatric symptoms and disorders. Changes in oxygenation of the brain will always result in alterations in behavior and mental status. Treating the symptoms can make the patient feel more comfortable, but it is crucial to establish the etiology of those symptoms, diagnose any underlying lung disease, and set up the appropriate referrals to provide the best, safest, evidence-based care to the patient.

References

Brownrigg, E. (2007). The patient's perspective. In D. Lynes (Ed.), *The management of COPD in primary and secondary care*. Liverpool, England: M&K Publishing.

Centers for Disease Control and Prevention. (2014). QuickStats: Average annual number of deaths and death rates from unintentional, non–fire-related carbon monoxide poisoning, by sex and age group—United States, 1999–2010. Retrieved from http://www.cdc.gov/mmwr/preview/mmwrhtml/mm6303a6.htm

Kewalramani, A., Bollinger, M. E., & Postolache, T. T. (2008). Asthma and mood disorders. *International Journal of Child Health and Human Development, 1*(2), 115–123.

Lieshout, R., & MacQueen, G. (2012) Relations between asthma and psychological distress: An old idea revisited. In H. Renz (Series Ed.), *Chemical*

Immunology and Allergy: Allergy and the nervous system (Vol. 98, pp. 1–13). Basel, Switzerland: Karger.

Sircar, K., Clower, J., Shin, M. K., Bailey, C., King, M., & Yip, R. (2015, September). Carbon monoxide poisoning deaths in the United States, 1999 to 2012. *American Journal of Emergency Medicine*, *33*(9), 1140–1145. doi:10.1016/j.ajem.2015.05.002. Epub 2015 May 13.

Tomaszewski, C. (2015). Carbon monoxide. In Hoffman, R. S., Howland, M. A., Lewin, N. A., Nelson, L. S., & Goldfrank, L. R. (Eds.), *Goldfrank's toxicologic emergencies* (10th ed., pp. 1689–1704). New York, NY: McGraw-Hill.

Website Resources: Online Sleep Apnea Questionnaires

BERLIN: http://sleepmedicine.com/files/Forms/berlin_questionnaire2.pdf

Epworth: http://sleepmedicine.com/files/Forms/epworth_sleepiness_scale.pdf

GASP: http://sleepmedicine.com/files/Forms/gasp_questionnaire.pdf

Preoperative Questionnaire: http://sleepmedicine.com/files/Forms/preoperative_questionnaire.pdf

STOP BANG: http://sleepmedicine.com/files/files/StopBang_Questionnaire.pdf

13

Medical Diagnosis and Symptom Sharing: Neurological Disease

In this chapter, you will learn:

- Symptoms that are shared between psychiatric disorders and neurological diseases
- Common symptoms that may be noted in patients with specific neurological disorders (traumatic brain injury, epilepsy, multiple sclerosis, and myasthenia gravis) who do not have a psychiatric diagnosis
- Neurological symptoms (acquired and hereditary) in presenting patients that can be mistaken for psychiatric symptoms
- Nursing actions to address patient's confounding symptoms

CONFOUNDING SYMPTOMS

It all starts with the brain. Whether a neurological disorder is genetic or acquired, our ability to negotiate the world we live in is compromised. Sometimes the disorder robs us of our ability to be mobile or takes away our memories; other times it silences or blinds us.

Neurological disorders are diseases that affect our brains and spinal cords and all the connecting nerves—in other words, our nervous systems. The disorders can have an electrical foundation (e.g., epilepsy), a biochemical foundation (e.g., multiple sclerosis), or a structural basis (e.g., a brain tumor). There are more than 600 neurological conditions that can have an impact on a person's health. Many co-occur with psychiatric disorders; others share symptoms that are grounded in the neurological condition itself. And some of the neurological disorders are outcomes of brain damage (e.g., traumatic brain injury [TBI]), which can cause brain dysfunction.

Among the more common neurological disorders with shared psychiatric symptoms are Parkinson's disease, multiple sclerosis (MS), epilepsy, stroke, brain tumors, postconcussion syndrome, chronic subdural hematoma, corticobasal degeneration (CBD), Creutzfeldt-Jakob disease, and transient global amnesia. Sometimes we refer to these diseases by their symptoms, such as spinal cord disorders, or movement disorders; however, it is the effects of the disease on the brain, spine, and nervous system that categorize them all as neurological disorders.

Nurses often are the ones to spend the most time with patients diagnosed with neurological conditions. Remember that a person's inability to speak does not indicate an inability to hear or understand. As a patient-centered profession, nursing must be guided by respect for the patient throughout our treatments and behaviors. If not, "unintentional labeling" of the patient can occur at the point of triage due to the patient's statement of chief complaint.

SHARED SYMPTOMS

The following symptoms are shared by both neurological and psychiatric disorders:

- Tingling or numbness
- Cognitive changes
- Headaches
- Depression
- Mood swings
- Personality changes
- Confusion
- Inappropriate affect (laughing or crying)
- Memory loss
- Unsteady gait
- Dementia

Our ability to take a thorough patient's history at the intake interview, and to recognize the impact of stress, can assist the patient to engage in a therapeutic alliance that will benefit both the patient and the delivery of health care. Often neurological diseases are seen as one disorder with similar neuromuscular symptoms; however, many of the symptoms that are presented during a hospitalization or doctor's visit can be mistaken for psychiatric disorders, especially if the underlying neurological condition has not yet been identified. As with metabolic and respiratory diseases, it is the specific observations made during the initial assessment that instruct our nursing practice interventions.

Initial Assessment

Assessment of a patient should include questions related to headaches, activities of daily living (ADL) function changes, numbness and pain, and fatigue. A Mini-Mental State Exam will provide information related to orientation, memory, level of consciousness, and cognitive status.

Fast Facts in the Spotlight

Neurological disorders can have an acute onset or be chronic and progressive. They can be vascular, electrical, structural, or chemical in nature, with presenting symptoms similar to psychiatric disorders. Establishing baseline vital signs and any history of neurological disease is imperative for proper response to a patient experiencing a neuro-emergency.

Any disease that affects a person's ability to navigate the everyday world is anxiety provoking. The inability to know whether you will be healthy today or suffer a seizure at work or school inserts a level of chronic tension. Patients with chronic neurological disorders learn how to adapt to the challenges and difficulties presented by their disease. Those with an acute-onset condition, such as a concussion disorder, may experience a traumatic response to the inability to perform activities as they did before. Emotional responses to an injury that may have long-term consequences on a person's ability to function are normal, and patients can be expected to go through stages of grief in adjusting to these events.

Stages of Grief

Neurological diseases can cause real and irreversible loss. In facing such loss, patients may demonstrate the stages of grief described by Kübler-Ross:

- Denial
- Anger
- Bargaining
- Depression
- Acceptance

The impact of this reality can cause symptoms of mood swings, depression, suicidal ideation, and explosive anger. Responding to the reality of one's own mortality is not a psychiatric disorder; it is a normal emotional response to loss. Supporting the person going through the stages of grief can help facilitate acceptance of the present reality and engage the patient in self-care.

This chapter focuses solely on neurological conditions that are not neurodegenerative in nature, as those disorders are discussed elsewhere (see Chapter 7).

COMMON NEUROLOGICAL DISEASES WITH SHARED PSYCHIATRIC SYMPTOMS

Chronic Traumatic Encephalopathy (Dementia Pugilistica) and Traumatic Brain Injury

Traumatic brain injury (TBI) has recently come into the spotlight with movies like *Concussion* that exposed the impact of brain injury on professional football players, and articles describing the impact of boxing on neurological functioning. According to the National Institutes of Health, TBI is an acquired injury to the brain from trauma, which causes brain damage. TBI can be mild, moderate, or severe, depending on the extent of the trauma and whether it is a one-time event or includes multiple events. Concussion and postconcussion syndromes are transient states of "neuronal and axonal derangement" (Gavett, Stern, & McKee, 2011). Not all TBIs are progressive, but recurrent trauma has been documented to cause a range of more severe problems that can progressively exacerbate memory, balance, and cognition.

Recognition of TBI, and the symptoms that ensue after multiple injuries, is not new. In fact, in 1928, the diagnosis of *dementia pugilistica* ("punch drunk") was identified in boxers. This condition, now termed "chronic traumatic encephalopathy" (CTE), reflects the cumulative, end-stage effects of multiple TBIs to the head and is 100% fatal. Brain alterations in CTE, identified through magnetic resonance imaging, include volume loss, diseased subcortical and periventricular white matter, insult to the cavum septum pellucidum, and overall reduction in brain mass (Ardila & Farlow, 2011; Gavett et al., 2011). The pathological brain changes in CTE are similar to those seen in Alzheimer's disease, and may even progress to parkinsonism. Patients who have CTE are also at increased risk of developing amyotrophic lateral sclerosis (ALS), Alzheimer's disease, and Parkinson's disease.

Prevalence and Incidence

Nearly 165,000 cases of CTE specifically related to boxing (dementia pugilistica) have been documented from 1990 to 2008 (Ardila & Farlow, 2011). The prevalence of all TBIs resulting in CTE is difficult to determine as diagnosis is based on postmortem brain tests. The mean age for presentation of symptoms of CTE is 42.8 years, and the severity of symptoms is related to the duration, intensity, and frequency of the brain insults (Gavett et al., 2011).

Presenting Psychiatric Symptoms

Headaches, loss of language abilities (having to search for words), ataxia, slurred speech, tremors, irritability, apathy, and being quick to anger

Other Symptoms

Balance issues, difficulties with executive function (i.e., planning and decision-making tasks), and short-term memory loss

Questions to Ask

- Do you play contact sports?
- Have you served in the military?
- Have you recently had head contact with someone, leaving you feeling as though you have "had your bell rung" or that you have "seen stars"?
- Have you ever been, or are you now, a victim of violence?

Interventions

- *RN*: Examine for any neurological changes, PERLA (pupils equal and reactive to light and accommodation), assess blood pressure, and alert the team if there is a potential that the patient is experiencing a postconcussion syndrome.
- *APRN*: Same as RN plus a full neurological workup.

Epilepsy (Seizure Disorder)

Seizures result from an alteration in the electrical activity in the brain, involving the neurochemical makeup and responsiveness of the brain. The cause is usually congenital, genetic, or the result of a brain injury or insult-like brain trauma or infection. The symptoms that manifest during a seizure reflect the area of the brain being affected by the seizure.

Table 13.1 describes signs and symptoms of various types of seizures. Common seizure disorders include temporal lobe epilepsy, and simple and complex partial seizures (see Table 13.2). "Epilepsy" is a common name for complex partial seizures.

Patients who had temporal lobe epilepsy were identified as having dream-like states, without the easily identified tonic–clonic, grand

Table 13.1

Types of Seizures

Type of seizure	Common signs and symptoms (Patient may . . .)
Grand mal/tonic–clonic	Shake violently, lose consciousness, and collapse
Tonic	Have muscles suddenly stiffen
Clonic	Exhibit jerking movements causing bilateral twitching movements
Atonic	Have a sudden and complete loss of muscle tone, causing a fall
Myoclonic	Exhibit sporadic shaking, usually bilateral. These patients might suddenly fall to the floor, grab, or throw objects near their reach.
Absence	Have no apparent, easily observable symptoms. Consciousness is lost for several seconds, with possible blank staring or blinking of the eyes.

Table 13.2

Types of Partial Seizures

Type of partial seizure	Presenting symptoms
Simple	
Motor	Head turning, twitching, jerking
Sensory	Sensory hallucinations: vision, hearing, smell, touch, tastes
Psychological	Changing emotional state, memory loss
Complex	Lip smacking, chewing movements, fidgeting, repetitive meaningless motions (finger tapping), coordinated but involuntary motions
Second-generation	Begins with patient appearing to maintain consciousness, then progresses to convulsions and loss of consciousness

mal seizure activity that is more commonly associated with the condition. These patients often report visual changes during the aura stage of the seizure, with objects appearing to be brighter, unreal, or somehow changed. The seizure may be simple or complex.

Simple Partial Seizures

During a simple partial seizure, the patient may not lose consciousness and instead may experience altered sense activation, emotional instability or lability, and loss of memory. During the complex partial seizure it is possible to see the same presenting symptoms as the simple partial seizure; however, there is the addition of an impairment of responsiveness and awareness. Partial seizures are called "partial" because they affect a specific part of the brain (focal seizures), so the variety of behavioral symptoms will be reflective of the brain region affected. Because patients can experience partial seizures without the loss of consciousness, it is possible for this condition to be mistaken for a psychiatric disorder.

Complex Partial Seizures

These seizures are characterized by three phases:

1. A prodromal period when the patient may experience an aura, which may include an increased sensitivity to lights, sounds, smells, tastes, or altered mental acuity, depending on the region of the brain affected.

2. Ictus, the seizure itself, which might be visible or not to the observer and may last a few seconds to a few minutes.
3. A postictal period, after the seizure is complete, during which the patient may complain of headache, sleepiness, nausea, depression, confusion, and exhaustion. The patient with complex partial seizures may have loss of memory related to the events surrounding the seizure.

Seizures that result from a serious medical condition will not present differently from epilepsy, so the patient must be evaluated for physical possible causes of the seizure to rule out brain tumor, drug or alcohol withdrawal, infection/fever, adverse drug reaction, endocrine or other metabolic disturbances, and drug-induced seizure activity.

Psychogenic, Non-Epileptic Seizures

Epileptic seizures, as previously mentioned, are caused by abnormal electrical brain activity. Some seizures, however, are not electrical abnormalities but rather are caused by a psychological conflict or disorder. They present very similarly and are involuntary, but their cause and treatments are very different. These seizures are psychogenic, non-epileptic seizures (ICD-10 F44.5), and they are related to acute stress and adjustment reactions. Patients can become very anxious due to experiencing these events and need to be reassured during the history taking and treatment of the underlying disorder (see Chapter 9).

Prevalence

Seizure disorders are the fourth most common neurological disorder affecting people of all ages, ethnicities, and genders (Shafer & Sirven, 2013).

Fast Facts in the Spotlight

Some famous people who have had epilepsy include Alexander the Great, Vincent Van Gogh, Michelangelo, Leonardo da Vinci, Sir Isaac Newton, Napoleon Bonaparte, Julius Caesar, Edgar Allan Poe, Dostoyevsky, Lewis Carroll, Agatha Christie, Charles Dickens, Richard Burton, Neil Young, and Danny Glover.

Source: "Famous People With Epilepsy," (n.d.).

Presenting Psychiatric Symptoms

Anxiety, depression, panic and fear, alternating laughing and crying not related to present situation, psychomotor retardation, ecstasy, and enhanced feelings of sexuality. Some patients may experience a behavioral arrest or sudden cessation of activity that makes them fall. Patients might also have transient hallucinations that affect their five senses, or an alteration in their ability to speak.

Other Symptoms

Abdominal pain or sensations, vertigo, dizziness, chest pain, palpitation, increased salivation, vomiting, repeated physical behaviors (automatisms) such as blinking, finger rolling, lip smacking, chewing motions, and involuntarily taking or throwing objects. People experiencing these symptoms appear to be unaware of their surroundings during the event.

Questions to Ask

- Have you ever had a seizure in the past?
- Do certain places or times make you feel this way (e.g., menstruation can be a trigger)?
- Do you ever "lose time" when you are doing something?
- Have you ever lost consciousness when you were doing something?
- Do you fall often without knowing why?
- Does anyone in your family have a seizure disorder?

Interventions

- *RN*: Examine for any neurological changes. Establish a safe environment, with the call bell in easy reach. Maintain safety precautions for possible fall risk.
- *APRN*: Same as RN plus full neurological workup.
- Referral to a neurologist.

Multiple Sclerosis

Multiple sclerosis (MS) is a disorder in which the body itself attacks and destroys the myelin that covers nerve cells. This demyelination interrupts the ability of the body's nervous system to communicate, resulting in various symptoms that affect cognition, movement, and emotional regulation. There is no known, identified cause of MS, nor is there presently a cure. MS is a chronic, progressive disease that has remissions and exacerbations.

Prevalence

MS is the most common of the central nervous system autoimmune disorders, which include myasthenia gravis (discussed next), Guillain-Barré syndrome, and limbic encephalitis (See Chapter 10, and Figure 10.4.). It is more common in women than in men, and symptom onset is usually between 20 and 50 years of age. A population-based examination of U.S. military veterans from the 1990–1991 Gulf War identified MS as a disease of interest. This is due to an increased incidence among Gulf War veterans when compared with nonveterans of the same age and sex. Whereas global prevalence of MS is 3 to 10 per 100,000, rates for Gulf War veterans were 9.6 per 100,000 for all cases and 24.7 for females—higher than any previously recorded incidence. The Gulf War study evaluated servicemen and -women from 1990 to 2007, with a mean age of 28 years (range: 19–50 years). Thus, some of those veterans are now men and women living with MS in their 60s (Wallin et al., 2012).

Presenting Psychiatric Symptoms

Mood disorder, often presenting with depressive symptoms, mania, anxiety, and pseudo-bulbar affect (alternating laughing and crying not related to, or appropriate for, the situation at hand); attention disturbances, memory loss, and decreased cognitive function; possible, though rare, psychotic episodes with delusions and hallucinations

Other Symptoms

Diplopia, transient loss of vision, easy fatigability, difficulties with bladder control, tingling, numbing sensations in the extremities, ataxia or other gait alterations, and motor difficulties resulting in tripping, stumbling, and falling

Questions to Ask

- Does anyone in your family have the same symptoms as you?
- Has anyone in your family been diagnosed with MS?
- Have you been having these symptoms a lot recently, or do they seem to come and go?

Interventions

- *RN*: Prepare the environment for a patient at increased risk of falls. Speak slowly and provide ample time for the patient to respond. Administer a mini-mental state exam.

- *APRN*: Same as RN plus full neurological workup.
- Referral to a neurologist.

Myasthenia Gravis

Myasthenia gravis (MG) is an autoimmune disorder that results in chronic neuromuscular disease. Antibodies interfere with the acetylcholine nicotinic postsynaptic receptors. Patients with MG have muscle weakness with rapid fatigue of voluntary muscle groups (i.e., those within the person's control), such as striated muscles. This disease is sometimes associated with tumors of the thymus gland and is often comorbid with other autoimmune diseases, such as thyroid disorders, lupus, and rheumatoid arthritis. There is an association between MG and long postoperative recovery from anesthesia.

Presenting Psychiatric Symptoms

Chronic complaints of muscle fatigue, depression, conversion disorder (emotional stress can precipitate MG symptoms); slowing of the cognitive process, and difficulty processing information

Other Symptoms

Blurred vision, diplopia, slurred speech, choking when eating, facial muscle weakness, shortness of breath, and respiratory failure

Questions to Ask

- How long have you felt this tired?
- Do you get tired when you laugh?
- Have you had this kind of feeling before?
- Have you ever had surgery and had a hard time recovering from the anesthesia?
- What kind of symptoms did you notice first?

Interventions

- *RN*: Provide ample time for questions and answers, allow for rest periods as the patient will fatigue very quickly, administer a mini-mental state exam, and prepare the environment for a patient at high risk for falls.
- *APRN*: Same as RN plus full neurological workup.
- Referral to a neurologist.

Table 13.3

Hypotheses nurses might make that could delay proper treatment for an organic disorder to the patient with a psychiatric disorder

- The patient has a history of psychiatric disease, therefore this admission must be related to the psychiatric disorder.
- The patient was brought into the psychiatric ED, therefore the patient only needs to be assessed for a psychiatric disorder.
- The patient is a youth, adolescent, teen, or young adult, so the presenting problem is probably due to a functional disorder.
- The patient is emotionally unstable, so any abnormalities in vital signs are probably secondary to the psychiatric problem or emotional dysregulation.

Nurses should be careful to avoid:
- Accepting a less-than-thorough history due to discomfort with interviewing a patient with a psychiatric disorder, or accepting only a history from the patient, if others are also available.
- Conducting a brief systems review, physical review, or psychiatric review, rather than a complete one.
- Neglecting to look over past and present medications and purpose for each.
- Abbreviating the intake interview to cover only mandatory questions, rather than investigating the facts and reserving judgment so as to make a nursing diagnosis based in the evidence, rather than in the possibly biased hypothesis.

TAKE-AWAY

Seizure disorders, MS, and MG are some of the more common neurological disorders that often present or coexist with psychiatric symptoms and disorders. These diseases all impair cognitive functioning and result in progressive deterioration when left untreated. A missed diagnosis can have serious consequences, delaying treatments that can sometimes halt the progression of the disease or improve the patient's quality of life. All missed diagnoses impact a patient's capacity for recovery; however, when a patient's symptoms are unintentionally or incorrectly labeled as being psychiatric in origin rather than neurological, the effects on the patient and family members may undermine confidence in, and adherence to, future treatments (see Table 13.3).

Further Reading

Gillig, P. M. (2013). Psychogenic nonepileptic seizures. *Innovations in Clinical Neuroscience, 10*(11–12), 15–18.

Levenson, R., Sturm, V., & Haase, C. (2014, March). Emotional and behavioral symptoms in neurodegenerative disease: A model for studying the neural bases of psychopathology. *Annual Review of Clinical Psychology, 10*, 581–601.

McKeon, A. (2013). Paraneoplastic and other autoimmune disorders of the central nervous system. *The Neurohospitalist, 3*(2), 53–64. doi:10.1177/1941874412453339

References

Ardila, A., & Farlow, M. (2011). Head trauma: Neurobehavioral aspects. Retrieved from http://www.medlink.com/article/dementia_pugilistica

Dorsey, S. (2002, September). Medical conditions that mimic psychiatric disease: A systematic approach for evaluation of patients who present with psychiatric symptomatology. *Emergency Medicine Reports*. Retrieved from https://www.ahcmedia.com/articles/109640-medical-conditions-that-mimic-psychiatric-disease-a-systematic-approach-for-evaluation-of-patients-who-present-with-psychiatric-symptomatology?trendmd-shared=0

Famous people with epilepsy. (n.d.). Retrieved from http://www.disabled-world.com/artman/publish/epilepsy-famous.shtml

Gavett, B. E., Stern, R. A., & McKee, A. C. (2011). Chronic traumatic encephalopathy: A potential late effect of sport-related concussive and subconcussive head trauma. *Clinics in Sports Medicine, 30*(1), 179–188. doi:10.1016/j.csm.2010.09.007

Shafer, P., & Sirven, J. (2013). Epilepsy statistics. *Epilepsy Foundation*. Retrieved from http://www.epilepsy.com/learn/epilepsy-statistics

Wallin, M., Culpepper, W., Coffman, P., Pulaski, S., Maloni, H., Mahan, C., . . . Kurtzke, J. (2012). The Gulf War era multiple sclerosis cohort: Age and incidence rates by race, sex and service. *Brain, 135*, 1778–1785.

Website Resources: Online Sleep Apnea Questionnaires

BERLIN: http://sleepmedicine.com/files/Forms/berlin_questionnaire2.pdf
Epworth: http://sleepmedicine.com/files/Forms/epworth_sleepiness_scale.pdf
GASP: http://sleepmedicine.com/files/Forms/gasp_questionnaire.pdf

IV

Addictive Disorders

14

Addictive Disorders, Substance Use, and Dependence

In this chapter, you will learn:

- What is meant by addictive disorders, substance use, abuse, and dependency
- Statistics related to addiction in the United States
- Barriers to treatment
- Terminology related to addiction disorders
- Criteria for an addiction disorder
- Designer/street drug names, routes, and presenting symptoms
- Nursing responsibilities and challenges when working with patients with substance use issues

THE SPECTRUM OF ADDICTIVE DISORDERS

Substance-related and addictive disorders include misuse of alcohol, caffeine, cannabis, hallucinogens, inhalants, opioids, sedatives, anxiolytics, stimulants, and tobacco. Nonsubstance-related addictive disorders include gambling, compulsive shopping, and other pathological patterns of behavioral engagement. Common to both the substance and nonsubstance addictive disorders is the component of craving, or undeniable desire to use, and engage in or with, the object of addiction.

Addiction is a brain-based disorder that impairs a person's ability to deny a normally suppressed behavioral response to an environment, substance, or stimulus. It is a complex brain disorder that involves circuitry alterations resulting in physiological changes, as well as alterations in cognition and behavior. *Relapse*, or a return to addictive behaviors after cessation, may reflect the intensity of the body to respond to underlying altered neurological circuitry changes. When the neurology of the brain is altered, there are changes in the brain's systems of reward, memory, and motivation. The drugs themselves affect the brain's neurocircuitry, increasing the likelihood of continuation of drug use by providing a sensation of reward for use and discomfort of withdrawal on cessation.

WHAT IS MEANT BY SUBSTANCE USE, SUBSTANCE ABUSE, AND DEPENDENCY?

Substance abuse exists on a continuum of engagement from abstinence to addition (see Table 14.1). *Substance use* becomes *substance abuse* when the individual's life becomes dysfunctional due to the repeated behaviors related to the substance. For most users, engagement is limited to experimentation and recreational use. Early substance use has been correlated to later development of substance abuse, due to multiple genetic and environmental risk factors (Richmond-Rakerd et al., 2016). A substance use disorder (SUD) exists when a situation of patterned abuse and dependency develops that results in chronic impairment or stress, which affects a person's physical and mental functioning and impacts his or her ability to function in society.

The diagnosis of mental illness cannot be determined by examining results from x-rays, blood tests, or urine tests. We don't learn of the presence of mental illness by using a sphygmomanometer, pulse oximeter, or thermometer. Diagnosis must be made on the basis of history and presenting symptoms, particularly symptoms that persist over time and change a person's ability to function in multiple aspects of daily life. Diagnosis of addictive disorders, like that of other mental disorders, depends on observation of a pathological response—but in this case, in the presence of the addicting stimulus.

Table 14.1

Continuum of Engagement: From Abstinence to Addiction

Not used	Experimentation (external pressure)	Recreation (external influence)	Abuse (patterned use)	Dependency/addiction (required)
Abstinence	Peer pressure	Using only in groups or	Increased importance	Craving
Never tried	Try once	socially	Decreased ability to meet	Seeking behavior
	Curiosity	Able to say no	responsibilities	Use all the time
	Choice to use to be socially	Self-regulated	Interferes with relationships	Utmost importance
	accepted	Control	Deciding factor in daily life	Need to have
	Control		Unable to control use	Withdrawal without use

STATISTICS OF ALCOHOL AND OTHER SUBSTANCE USE IN THE UNITED STATES

Alcohol

According to the National Institute on Alcohol Abuse and Alcoholism (NIAAA), in 2014 almost 90% of adults aged 18 years or older used alcohol. About 25% of those surveyed revealed that they had engaged in binge drinking (heavy drinking) in the month before the survey. In 2015, alcohol use disorder was present in about 6.2% of U.S. adults, or 15.1 million adults in all (Substance Abuse and Mental Health Services Administration [SAMHSA], 2015c). These statistics have devastating implications for individuals and society. Thirty-one percent of all driving fatalities are attributed to alcohol impairment (NIAAA, 2017). Problems related to alcohol misuse carry a $249 billion price tag in the United States (Sacks, Gonzales, Bouchery, Tomedi, & Brewer, 2010).

Alcohol Abuse and Dependence Among Specific Populations

Examining specific groups of users reveals that full-time college students make up the greatest number of drinkers in their age group. About 60% of college students report drinking alcohol, with almost 38% indicating engagement in binge drinking (five or more drinks for males, four or more drinks for females in about 2 hours). More than 12% engage in alcohol consumption that indicates abuse or dependency (NIAAA, 2017). Figure 14.1 graphs lifetime rates of alcohol abuse and dependence by ethnicity.

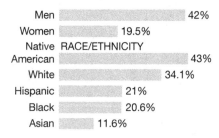

Percentage of Americans suffering from alcohol abuse or dependence in their lifetime

Men	42%
Women	19.5%
Native American	RACE/ETHNICITY — 43%
White	34.1%
Hispanic	21%
Black	20.6%
Asian	11.6%

Figure 14.1 Alcohol abuse and dependence by ethnicity. *Source: SAMHSA (2014).*

Alcohol Abuse and Dependence by Age of First Use

Age of first use is an important factor when working with patients with SUDs. The NIAAA (2017) notes that the earlier the first use of alcohol, for example, the higher the likelihood of drug abuse and dependence.

Prevalence of Drinking
Statistics from the National Survey on Drug Use and Health (NSDUH) indicate that more than 86% of those 18 years of age or older reported that they drank alcohol "at some point in their lifetime"; just over 70% reported that they drank in the past year; and 56% reported that they drank in the past month (SAMHSA, 2015a).

Prevalence of Heavy and Binge Drinking
Additionally, according to the 2015 NSDUH, approximately 7% of Americans over 18 had engaged in heavy alcohol use during the month preceding the survey, and almost 27% reported binge drinking. Just over 15 million adults (9.8% of males, 5.3% of females) in the United States reported having an alcohol use disorder (AUD), with only 1.3 million receiving treatment (8.3% of those requiring treatment).

Prevalence of Youth (Ages 12 to 17 Years) Use of Alcohol
Approximately 623,000 American adolescents have an AUD, according to the 2015 NSDUH statistics, with 37,000 receiving some treatment (SAMHSA, 2015b).

Consequences of Alcohol Use
Adolescent alcohol use could interfere with normal brain development, and increases the risk of developing an AUD later in life (Richmond-Rakerd et al., 2016; Tapert, Caldwell, & Burke, n.d.). Underage drinking contributes to a range of acute consequences, which include injuries, sexual assaults, and even deaths. Alcohol deaths are the fourth leading cause of preventable deaths in the United States, with 88,000 alcohol-related deaths annually (Mokdad, Marks, Stroup, & Gerberding, 2004; NIAAA, 2017).

Illicit Drug and Other Substance Use

In the month before taking the national SAMHSA's survey in 2014, more than 10% of Americans aged 12 years and older used an illicit drug (see Figure 14.2). Marijuana, the most commonly listed illicit

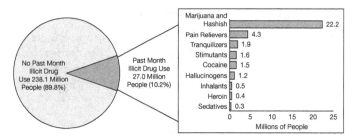

Figure 14.2 Numbers of past-month illicit drug users among people aged 12 or older: 2014. *Source: Center for Behavioral Health Statistics and Quality (2015).*

Note: Estimated numbers of people refer to people aged 12 or older in the civilian, noninstitutionalized population in the United States. The numbers do not sum to the total population of the United States because the population for NSDUH does not include people aged 11 years old or younger, people with no fixed household address (e.g., homeless of transient people not in shelters), active-duty military personnel, and residents of institutional group quarters, such as correctional facilities, nursing homes, mental institutions, and long-term hospitals.

Note: The estimated numbers of current users of different illicit drugs are not mutually exclusive because people could have used more than one type of illicit drug in the past month.

substance, showed a rise in use in comparison from 2002 to 2013. Use of nonmedical pain relievers was the second most common illicit drug use (1.6%), with usage statistics similar to 2013, but lower than usage from 2002 to 2012. Eight percent of Americans 12 years of age or older (21.5 million) met the criteria for an SUD—a definition that includes alcoholism (SAMHSA, 2014). Approximately 3% of all U.S. adults met criteria for both existing mental illness and an SUD, which is referred to as "co-occurring mental illness and substance use disorder," or "dual diagnosis."

BARRIERS TO TREATMENT

Symptoms of psychiatric disorders, especially when they occur in childhood, adolescence, or early adulthood are alarming to the individual and family, and often to the community as well. Fear of being labeled "crazy" and thoughts of the stereotypical media rendition of an insane person can be barriers to treatment that either delay or prevent effective interventions from occurring.

Adolescence and young adulthood are natural ages for experimentation with drugs, alcohol, sex, and other risky behaviors. Brain development at this stage of life is associated with a sense of invulnerability. Although different parts of the brain mature at different times, the years between 13 and 24 constitute the second significant period of brain growth in an individual's life. There is a period of synaptic growth in the area of executive function (prefrontal cortex) just prior to puberty, then a "pruning" or trimming back of synapses during the adolescent years. This is also a time when the cerebellum experiences rapid changes. Even excluding any psychiatric diagnosis, these years are filled with changes in the adolescent's family role, personal appearance, and sexual development. Transient anxiety, depression, social withdrawal, and increased desire for experimentation are normal, but also extremely challenging to emotional self-regulation.

The harmful effects of biased nomenclature when considering substance use cannot be overstated. Use of the correct words, and understanding their meaning, can remove one of the barriers to providing safe and effective treatment to the person with an SUD (see Table 14.2). If dependence carries with it the judgment that the person is an "addict"—a term that can elicit an often media-driven image of a

Table 14.2

Terminology Related to Addiction Disorders

Addiction	Chronic, compulsive, relapsing disorder in which the individual craves, seeks, and engages in using behaviors despite negative consequences and possible irreversible brain alteration
Tolerance	Increased resistance to initial "high" in which more of the substance is required to achieve desired effects; may indicate physical dependence
Withdrawal	Rapid decrease in levels of substance after chronic use; could result from lack of access to the drug or use of a reversal agent such as naloxone HCl (Narcan); *may indicate a medical emergency*
Detoxification	Period of withdrawing drugs, alcohol, and other addictive substances from the body; *can present a medical emergency*
Poly drug use	Use of two or more substances concurrently (e.g., marijuana, cocaine, and alcohol)
Prescription drug abuse	Using prescribed medications without a prescription or other than prescribed; also referred to as "nonmedical use"

Source: www.drugabuse.gov/publications/media-guide/glossary

stereotypical bum or druggie—the patient will be reluctant to share personal information with you. If a patient has sought care for a broken arm, and the nursing staff's determination is that this patient is an addict, it is quite possible that the amount of pain medication to be provided will not be sufficient to reduce the real, existing pain that exposes the patient to suffering. If the patient does not share that he or she has an existing SUD diagnosis, it is also possible that withdrawal might occur at some time during treatment.

Fast Facts in the Spotlight

More than 3% of adults and 1.4% of adolescents in the United States have a dual diagnosis. Many people seeking medical care for a physical ailment (common cold, injury, stomach ailments, etc.) will not share with the nurse that they also have mental illness and SUDs. Establishing a therapeutic relationship that creates a safe, nonjudgmental environment can assist the nurse in identifying any coexisting diagnosis that could impact safe, effective treatment of the presenting illness.

CRITERIA FOR AN ADDICTION DISORDER

The criteria for diagnosing addiction disorders, regardless of the substances or behavior being addressed, are the same. The first requirement is for the health care professional to identify the patterned behavior of use, establishing frequency, intensity, and persistence regardless of consequence. This can be done through the initial questions posed by the nurse during the interview. When it is established that the patient is engaging in a repeated pattern of problematic behavior that includes craving, seeking, and an inability to resist the behavior despite consequences, the health care professional should seek to identify the substance and pose direct substance-specific questions. Signs and symptoms of common SUDs are summarized in Table 14.3.

COMMON DESIGNER DRUGS

Designer drugs, also known as "street," "synthetic," or "club" drugs, are manufactured in illegal laboratories, and are created to chemically

Table 14.3

Signs and Symptoms of Common Substance Use Disorders

Disorder definition	Signs and symptoms of use	Signs and symptoms of withdrawal
Alcohol Use Disorder Patterned use of alcohol to excess despite the consequences; inability to cut back or stop, spending time seeking and obtaining alcohol or recovering from overuse of alcohol, tending to alcohol need above other responsibilities (work, family, community), use despite risk of harm, and withdrawal symptoms in the absence of use	Ataxia/unsteady gait, slurred speech, difficulty remembering things, uncoordinated movements, and stupor (or coma)	Stage 1: Anxiety, insomnia, tremors, depression, mood swings Stage 2: Increase in temperature, respirations, and BP; confusion, irritability, and mood changes Stage 3: Hallucinations, seizures, confusion, agitation and fever
Caffeine Use Disorder Patterned use of caffeine and substances with caffeine despite significant impact on physical and psychological functioning	Psychomotor agitation, stomach and other GI problems, nervousness, insomnia, uncontrolled muscle twitching, and tachycardia (often with cardiac arrhythmias)	Headache, inability or difficulty focusing concentration, flu-like symptoms, depression, and fatigue
Cannabis Use Disorder Patterned use of marijuana that increases over time (tolerance) with a demonstrated inability to cut back on use; indications of cravings, seeking behaviors, and continued use of cannabis despite knowledge of problems related to use on personal and professional relationships; cannabis use becomes more important than other responsibilities and will be pursued even when risk of harm to self and others is great	Red, bloodshot eyes in the absence of conjunctivitis; hunger; possible tachycardia; thirst; euphoric attitude; and possible hallucinations	Nervousness, anxiety, decreased appetite, irritability, possible stomach aches, flu-like symptoms, and restlessness

(continued)

Table 14.3

Signs and Symptoms of Common Substance Use Disorders (*continued*)		
Disorder definition	**Signs and symptoms of use**	**Signs and symptoms of withdrawal**
Hallucinogen Use Disorder Harmful, patterned use of hallucinogens (e.g., phencyclidine) despite risks of harm to self or others, interference in social interactions, and use in hazardous situations; presence of cravings, seeking behaviors, and tolerance to substance	Hallucinations, nystagmus, ataxia, numbness, dilated pupils, sweating, tremors, and incoordination	Flashbacks of a hallucinogenic state even many years after use; abrupt cessation of the drugs may cause diarrhea and chills
Inhalant Use Disorder Patterned use of inhalants despite impairment and distress due to use; increasing frequency of use, cravings, and seeking behaviors; continued use despite risks, with increasing amounts of inhalant used during usage period (tolerance)	Slurred speech, ataxia, incoordination, dizziness, lethargy, depressed reflexes, tremors, and euphoria	Sweating, insomnia, tachycardia, nausea, vomiting tremors, seizures
Opioid Use Disorder Patterned use of opioids despite impairment of ability to engage in activities of daily living or relationships with others, and risk to emotional and physical health; increasing tolerance to opioids, requiring increasing doses; presence of cravings; seeking and using behaviors; continued use with a disregard for risks to self and others	Pinpoint pupils, memory impairment, drowsiness, slurred speech, and possible perceptual disturbances, including hallucinations	Depression, flu-like symptoms, insomnia, nausea and vomiting, yawning, diarrhea, pupil dilation, and fever

(*continued*)

Table 14.3

Signs and Symptoms of Common Substance Use Disorders (*continued*)		
Disorder definition	Signs and symptoms of use	Signs and symptoms of withdrawal
CNS Depressant Use Disorder Patterned and problem-producing use of CNS depressants (anxiolytics, hypnotics, and sedatives) that interferes with engagement in activities of daily living; impairment in personal and professional functioning due to use, with behaviors of craving, seeking, and obtaining CNS depressants	Impaired cognitions, unsteady gait, slurred speech, incoordination, and stupor	Tremors, nausea, vomiting, psychomotor agitation, hallucinations, insomnia, anxiety, and seizures

BP, blood pressure; CNS, central nervous system; GI, gastrointestinal.

mimic existing illicit drugs. Designer drugs are usually stronger and more lethal than the street drugs they seek to imitate. One of the earliest examples of a designer drug is heroin, which was a chemically altered form of the morphine alkaloid, which originated from the opium poppy. Table 14.4 lists common designer drugs. The production of these drugs is not regulated, and the initial drug is usually combined with other drugs, including over-the-counter, prescription, and other illegal drugs. Some of these drugs have therapeutic uses when prescribed by a health care provider and used as directed.

NURSING CHALLENGES AND RESPONSIBILITIES WHEN WORKING WITH PATIENTS WHO HAVE SUBSTANCE USE ISSUES

Some patients might be seeking care because they *want* to stop using, but many more may become your patient due to a medical incident that has interrupted their drug use. The nurse's responsibility to

Table 14.4

Common Designer Drugs

Drug name (street names)	Composition and route	Symptoms of use
Ecstasy	In 2011, 2.5 million ED visits were associated with drug misuse or abuse (Services Substance Abuse and Mental Health Services Administration 2013)	Hypertension, anxiety, blurred vision, aggression, arrhythmia, increased body temperature, teeth grinding and abdominal cramping
K-2 Spice	Synthetic cannabinoids; industrial chemicals sprayed on dried leaves to look like cannabis	Zombie-like behavior, seizures, anxiety, agitation, vomiting, hallucinations, paranoia, and vomiting
Ketamine	Anesthetic drug, taken IM, orally, and dissolved in liquid (often alcohol); a date rape drug	Euphoria, dizziness, sense of floating, sedation, dissociation, and amnesia
GHB Liquid X, Liquid Ecstasy, Georgia Home Boy, Oop, Gamma-Oh, Grievous Bodily Harm, Mils, G, Liquid G, Fantasy, others	CNS depressant; originally a drug for treating narcolepsy (sodium oxylate); taken orally and mixed in liquid; a date rape drug	Euphoria, increased sex drive, tranquility, loss of consciousness, nausea, hallucinations, coma, and amnesia; can cause vomiting during sleep/aspiration
Rohypnol (flunitrazepam) Forget-Me drug, Roches, Roofies, Ruffles, others	Intermediate-acting benzodiazepine; originally used to treat insomnia and as an anesthetic for presurgical prep; a date rape drug	Sedation, muscle relaxation, amnesia, slurred speech, dizziness, drowsiness, GI disturbances
Methamphetamine Meth, Crystal, Chalk, and Ice	As a prescription drug used to treat ADD and ADHD; increases dopamine levels; taken orally, snorted, in liquid and injected	Energetic, talkative, anxious, insomnia, confusion, weight loss, euphoria, tachycardia, increased BP

(continued)

Table 14.4

Common Designer Drugs (*continued*)

Drug name (street names)	Composition and route	Symptoms of use
Bath Salts (PABS) Flakka, Ivory Wave, Vanilla Sky, Cloud Nine, Blue Silk, Purple Sky, Bliss, Purple Wave, Red Dove, Zoom, Bloom, Ocean Snow, Lunar Wave, White Lightening, Scarface, Hurricane Charlie, others	CNS stimulants, related to MDMA; "legal cocaine," usually snorted; highly addictive	Delusional states

ADD, attention deficit disorder; ADHD, attention deficit hyperactivity disorder; BP, blood pressure; CNS, central nervous system; GHB, gamma hydroxybutyrate; GI, gastrointestinal; IM, intramuscular; MDMA, 3,4-methylenedioxymethamphetamine; PABS, psychoactive bath salts.

patients with an addiction disorder is first and foremost to keep them safe and provide effective, evidence-based, nonjudgmental care.

Providing Safe, Effective, and Nonjudgmental Care

Learning that a patient has an SUD usually occurs through careful observation, questioning, and development of a therapeutic alliance. Your patient might be a substance abuser who is pregnant; a teen who is hallucinating after taking a "designer drug"; a college student with alcohol and food poisoning; a newborn with cocaine addiction; or an elderly retired nurse with the signs of congestive heart failure, who is alcohol dependent. Your first responsibility is to use your experience and education to accurately determine what is going on with the patient and determine what the priority is for that person's well-being. No matter what unit you work on or what your specialty in nursing, you will at some time be caring for patients with SUDs. Identifying your own personal biases and feelings toward the use of both legal and illegal addictive substances, and learning strategies to remain mindful of the needs of the patient in distress, can assist you to provide the best nursing care that results in positive patient outcomes.

Questions to Ask

The questions should seek to establish the existence of the SUD:

- What substance, including alcohol and drugs, have you used in the past? (Do you regularly drink or use drugs?)
- Are you using any substances presently?
- When was the last time you used?
- Are you in treatment for an addiction? If so, what is your addiction, and what is the treatment you have been receiving?

Further Reading

Drug Enforcement Administration Museum & Visitors Center. (n.d.). Cannabis, coca & poppy: Nature's addictive plants. Retrieved from https://www.deamuseum.org/ccp

Naussbaum, A. (2013). *The pocket guide to the DSM-5 diagnostic exam.* Arlington, VA: American Psychiatric Publishing.

Stahl, S., & Grady. M. (2012). *Stahl's illustrated substance use and impulsive disorders.* Cambridge, UK: Cambridge University Press.

References

Center for Behavioral Health Statistics and Quality. (2015). *Behavioral health trends in the United States: Results from the 2014 National Survey on Drug Use and Health.* Retrieved from http://www.samhsa.gov/data/sites/default/files/NSDUH-FRR1-2014/NSDUH-FRR1-2014.pdf

Mokdad, A. H., Marks, J. S., Stroup, D. F., & Gerberding, J. L. (2004). Actual causes of death in the United States 2000. *Journal of the American Medical Association, 291*(10), 1238–1245.

National Institute on Alcohol Abuse and Alcoholism. (2017). Alcohol facts and statistics. Retrieved from https://www.niaaa.nih.gov/alcohol-health/overview-alcohol-consumption/alcohol-facts-and-statistics

Richmond-Rakerd, L. S., Slutske, W. S., Lynskey, M. T., Agrawal, A., Madden, P. A., Bucholz, K. K., . . . Martin, N. G. (2016). Age at first use and later substance use disorder: Shared genetic and environmental pathways for nicotine, alcohol, and cannabis. *Journal of Abnormal Psychology, 125*(7), 946–959. doi:10.1037/abn0000191

Sacks, J. J., Gonzales, K. R., Bouchery, E. E., Tomedi, L. E., & Brewer, R. D. (2010). 2010 national and state costs of excessive alcohol consumption. *American Journal of Preventive Medicine 49*(5), e73–e79.

Substance Abuse and Mental Health Services Administration. (2013). Drug abuse warning network, 2011: National estimates of drug-related emergency department visits (HHS Publication No. [SMA] 13-4760, DAWN

Series D-39). Retrieved from: https://www.samhsa.gov/data/sites/default/files/DAWN2k11ED/DAWN2k11ED/DAWN2k11ED.pdf

Substance Abuse and Mental Health Services Administration. (2014). Results from the 2013 National Survey on Drug Use and Health: Summary of national findings. Retrieved from http://www.samhsa.gov/data/sites/default/files/NSDUHresultsPDFWHTML2013/Web/NSDUHresults2013.htm

Substance Abuse and Mental Health Services Administration. (2015a). Results from the 2015 National Survey on Drug Use and Health: Table 6.84B—Tobacco product and alcohol use in past month among persons aged 18 to 22, by college enrollment status: Percentages, 2014 and 2015. Retrieved from https://www.samhsa.gov/data/sites/default/files/NSDUH-DetTabs-2015/NSDUH-DetTabs-2015/NSDUH-DetTabs-2015.htm#tab6-84b

Substance Abuse and Mental Health Services Administration. (2015b). Results from the 2015 National Survey on Drug Use and Health: Table 2.41B—Alcohol use in lifetime, past year, and past month among persons aged 12 or older, by demographic characteristics: Percentages, 2014 and 2015. Retrieved from https://www.samhsa.gov/data/sites/default/files/NSDUH-DetTabs-2015/NSDUH-DetTabs-2015/NSDUH-DetTabs-2015.htm#tab2-41b

Substance Abuse and Mental Health Services Administration. (2015c). Results from the 2015 National Survey on Drug Use and Health: Table 5.6A—Substance use disorder in past year among persons aged 18 or older, by demographic characteristics: Numbers in thousands, 2014 and 2015. Retrieved from https://www.samhsa.gov/data/sites/default/files/NSDUH-DetTabs-2015/NSDUH-DetTabs-2015/NSDUH-DetTabs-2015.htm#tab5-6a

Tapert, S., Caldwell, L., & Burke, C. (n.d.). Alcohol and the adolescent brain—Human studies. Retrieved from https://pubs.niaaa.nih.gov/publications/arh284/205-212.htm

15

Dual Diagnosis: Mental Illness and Substance Use Disorder

In this chapter, you will learn:

- What is meant by dual diagnosis
- Statistics related to dual diagnosis in the United States
- Theories of causation in dual diagnosis
- Issues surrounding the opioid epidemic and dual diagnosis
- Nursing challenges and responsibilities when working with persons with dual diagnosis

Patients with dual diagnosis, or co-occurring mental illness and a substance use disorder (SUD), present a special challenge to health care providers. To put this in a medically framed perspective, consider the challenges a nurse faces when caring for a patient who has multiple sclerosis (MS) and transient ischemic attacks (TIAs). It would be difficult to tease out which symptoms were due to the MS and which reflected the TIA. But the health care team would be able to request diagnostic tests, which indicate when a patient is experiencing TIAs, and could evaluate specific criteria (including damage to the central nervous system [CNS]), which form the basis for an MS diagnosis.

It is much more difficult to differentiate key findings related to one disorder versus another when evaluating a patient with dual diagnosis of a mental illness and an SUD. When we are caring for a patient with mental illness, there is no lab test to provide key indications. Determining the existence of an SUD relies on the patient's self-report, or the corroboration by others who are reliable historians of the patient's behaviors. Each of the two categories in dual diagnosis—mental illness and SUD—is quite large and carries its own sets of criteria, symptoms, interventions, and stigma. Nearly 8 million Americans are estimated to have a dual diagnosis (see Figure 15.1).

Treatment of dual diagnosis began in the 1980s when mental health practitioners determined that providing separate treatments was not conducive to patient recovery. This approach increased interdisciplinary collaboration and created therapeutic milieus where patients could receive treatment for their substance disorders and psychiatric disorders concurrently. This supportive alliance increases patients' access to multiple providers and continuity of care. Despite this approach, many patients with dual diagnosis are not receiving the care needed to enter into recovery.

Consider the myriad mental illnesses, from mild attention deficit disorder to psychosis, and the diverse set of symptoms for each. *Any mental illness* (AMI) is differentiated from *serious mental illness* (SMI) in the SAMHSA statistical reports. When examining the substance use aspect of dual diagnosis, there are numerous substances, each

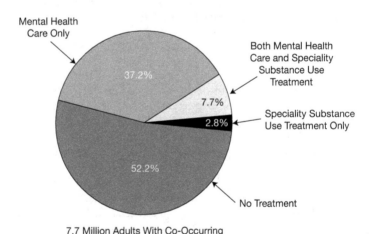

Mental Health Care Only

Both Mental Health Care and Speciality Substance Use Treatment

37.2%

7.7%

2.8%

Speciality Substance Use Treatment Only

52.2%

No Treatment

7.7 Million Adults With Co-Occurring Mental Illness and Substance Use Disorders

Figure 15.1 Adults with co-occurring mental illness and substance abuse disorders. *Source: Substance Abuse and Mental Health Services Administration ([SAMHSA], 2014).*

with specific symptoms and nursing interventions. What this diagnosis reveals to the health care community is the important biopsychosocial aspect of dual diagnosis, the diversity of patients and illnesses, and the need for a comprehensive recovery treatment model.

The increased difficulty of determining whether a patient has a dual diagnosis, however, does not reduce or change the responsibilities of the nurse to provide individualized, safe, effective, evidence-based care. The special challenge that this diagnosis presents includes the threat that the untreated second diagnosis (either SUD or mental illness) can serve as a trigger that can reverse treatment and return the patient to illness. Treating only the SUD or only the mental illness still leaves the patient at high risk for relapse.

STATISTICS

Adults

The SAMHSA 2014 behavioral health trends survey identified that almost 40% of the 7.9 million Americans with an SUD had a co-occurring mental illness, compared with only 16% of those without an SUD. Adults between the ages of 26 and 49 years accounted for the greatest number of those diagnosed with SUD and AMI (42.7%). This is in contrast to the 29.3% of 18- to 25-year-olds who presented with an AMI and were subsequently diagnosed with a co-occurring SUD. SAMHSA estimates that 21.5 million people, aged 12 and older, had an SUD in 2014 (see Figure 15.2).

Children and Adolescents

SAMHSA estimates that in 2014, about 271,000 (1.1%) of American adolescents had a co-occurring SUD and major depressive episode. Substance use has been linked to the diagnosis of major depressive disorder, with illicit drug use, alcohol use, and cigarette consumption noted in the 12- to 17-year-old patients who experienced a major depressive episode. Over 12% of adolescents diagnosed with a major depressive event had a co-occurring SUD.

THEORIES OF CAUSATION

Various theories have sought to explain the increased use of drugs by the mentally ill. Some of the more common are summarized

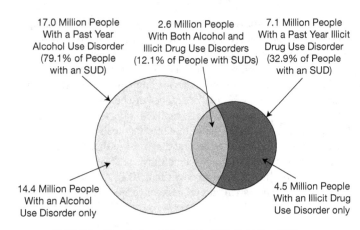

17.0 Million People With a Past Year Alcohol Use Disorder (79.1% of People with an SUD)

2.6 Million People With Both Alcohol and Illicit Drug Use Disorders (12.1% of People with SUDs)

7.1 Million People With a Past Year Illicit Drug Use Disorder (32.9% of People with an SUD)

14.4 Million People With an Alcohol Use Disorder only

4.5 Million People With an Illicit Drug Use Disorder only

21.5 Million People Aged 12 or Older With Past Year SUDs

Figure 15.2 Number of people aged 12 or older with past-year SUDs. *Source: Center for Behavioral Health Statistics and Quality (2015).*

SUD, substance use disorder.

here. None is definitive, and no studies have clarified the causal effect of use of drugs on mental health or mental health on the use of drugs. What we know, however, is that there is a relationship between the two.

Multiple Risk Theory

This theory proposes that access to drugs and exposure to others using drugs, without a structured environment that provides emotional support, can increase the possibility of substance use in a person with an existing mental illness. Social isolation as well as socioeconomic factors that can impact emotional well-being are factored into this theory.

Substance Causality Theory

This theory posits that substances with psychopharmacological and hallucinogenic properties can, with use, and will, with abuse, lead to the development of mental illness—specifically psychosis. Some drugs that fall into this category are cannabis, phencyclidine (PCP), ecstasy, LSD and psilocybin, mescaline, and peyote. There has been no proof to substantiate this theory; further, despite the increased use of cannabis with legalization, there has been no significant change in the rate of psychosis.

Self-Medication Theory

This theory suggests that people with mental illness will self-medicate themselves in order to relieve their distressing symptoms. The medication or substance that is chosen usually is specific to the negative signs of the underlying mental illness. Examples might include a person who is depressed and starts to use cocaine or amphetamines to feel "up," or a person with mania who damps down symptoms by using alcohol, barbiturates, or other CNS depressants. This theory is very similar to the *alleviation of dysphoria theory,* which suggests that self-medication is used to combat a poor self-image.

THE OPIOID EPIDEMIC AND DUAL DIAGNOSIS

Abuse of opioids is an epidemic in the United States, with drug overdose identified as the current leading cause of injury and death (U.S. Department of Health and Human Services [HHS], 2016). The Opioid Epidemic fact sheet developed by the U.S. HHS (see Website Resources at the end of this chapter) reflects the enormity of the problem, the financial impact on the government, the extreme challenges it places on providing care in emergency departments and inpatient wards, and the loss of life.

Opioids have been used by humans for millennia, and used medicinally to treat pain, diarrhea, and coughing. The drugs in this category are highly effective as painkillers. Global prescriptions for opioids in 1991 were around 76 million, which increased to 207 million in 2013. The largest global consumer of these prescribed medications was the United States, accounting for 100% of the prescribed hydrocodone (Vicodan) and over 80% of the oxycodone (Percocet). As the number of prescriptions increased, so did the number of overdose deaths (Volkow, 2014). More than 240 million opioid prescriptions were written in 2014, and approximately 650,000 opioid prescriptions were dispensed on an average day in 2015 (HHS, 2015). Concurrent with the increase in sales has been an increase in overdoses from opioids, including heroin. The connection between the two is illustrated by the following scenario: A person might begin using a prescribed painkiller, such as oxycodone (OxyContin or Percocet), after a tooth extraction or minor surgical procedure, but if dependency occurs and the prescription is no longer available, the individual will seek a comparable (and often less expensive) street replacement. Dart et al. (2015) demonstrated that there is a direct correlation between the prescribing of legitimate opioids, the distribution of illegal opioids, and the negative associated outcomes of abuse of opioids. Between 2004 and 2011, opioid-related medical emergencies increased 183%.

Not everyone who is prescribed an opioid will go on to develop an SUD; however between 2002 and 2011, 25 million Americans started to use nonprescription opioids (Dart et al., 2015). Multiple factors—including genetics, access, cost, social environment, emotional well-being, route of administration, and preexisting mental illness—are involved in susceptibility to addiction. Introduction, access, and continued use of a powerful opioid are dangerous for any brain.

Populations at High Risk

- People diagnosed with posttraumatic stress disorder (PTSD)
- People belonging to gender identity groups: lesbian, gay, bisexual, transgender, and questioning (LGBTQ)
- Children and adult children of alcoholics, drug addicts, and the chronically mentally ill

NURSING CHALLENGES AND RESPONSIBILITIES WHEN WORKING WITH PATIENTS WHO HAVE A DUAL DIAGNOSIS

Words Matter: Providing a Safe, Nonjudgmental Environment

Often it is the nurse who establishes a rapport with the patient and family/significant others through which discussion of a possible dual diagnosis is encouraged. Finding the words that convey support and understanding, rather than judgment and stigma, may be the most important elements of the nurse's first encounter with the patient and family—perhaps the only opportunity the individual will have to move toward recovery. Using words such as "junkie," when speaking of a person with an addiction, or referring to a "dirty" lab result rather than a positive lab result, can convey a perception of moral superiority on the part of the nurse, which can cut off the possibility of a therapeutic alliance. Patients with a dual diagnosis are sometimes homeless, may be paranoid, and are often very sick people; they need the attention and good care that can help them start on a path toward recovery.

Questions to Ask

The questions should seek to establish the existence of both the mental illness and the SUD:

- Have you ever been treated by a psychiatrist, psychologist, psychiatric nurse practitioner or other mental health provider?
- Are you presently under the care of a psychiatrist, nurse practitioner, or mental health provider for mental health reasons?
- Have you ever been told you have a mental or psychiatric illness?
- Do you take any medications now? Can I get a list of them? (Look for psychotropic drugs.)
- Do you take any drugs that are not medically prescribed for you?
- Do you regularly use drugs, cigarettes, or alcohol? How frequently do you use?
- How much alcohol (drugs, cigarettes) do you use?
- Do you ingest, snort, smoke, or shoot any drugs?

Treatment Priorities for a Patient With Dual Diagnosis

A patient who has a dual diagnosis requires treatment for the substance use problem (detoxification) first, and then ongoing therapy for the SUD and mental illness. Every nurse can play an enormous role in assisting patients to access the help they need, through establishing a respectful atmosphere where psycho-education can take place. Explaining the importance of receiving treatment for both disorders can help the patient begin the journey toward recovery.

Support Groups

Nurses can provide patients with referrals to support groups where, in a supportive environment, they will be able to meet others with similar diagnoses.

Evidence-Based Strategies for Assessing and Managing Addictions and Dual Diagnosis

Assessment

Screening tools can assist the nurse to examine the likelihood that a dual diagnosis (SUD and mental illness) exists. They include:

- CAGE: C—cut down, A—annoyed, G—guilty, E—eye opener
- AUDIT: Alcohol, Use Disorder, Identification Test
- ASSIST: Alcohol, Smoking, Substance Involvement Screening Test
- DAST: Drug Abuse Screening Test

Screening guides for dual diagnosis are available on the Internet though different initiatives. A comprehensive toolkit that is available online is listed at the end of this chapter (see Croton, 2007, under Website Resources).

Treatment

A comprehensive PowerPoint presentation on treating the patient with co-occurring addiction and mental health disorders, developed by D. Koiula, a registered nurse, can be accessed online (see Website Resources).

TAKE-AWAY

Dual diagnosis, or the presence of a mental illness and a concurrent SUD, can be present in patients in every specialty of nursing from maternity to geriatrics. Understanding the life challenges these patients face on a daily basis; determining how to provide a safe, non-judgmental environment; and utilizing evidence-based measures to screen, treat, or refer them to specialists can change the course of their recovery.

Further Reading

Anthony, J. C., & Helzer, J. E. (1991). Syndromes of drug abuse and dependence. In L. N. Robins & D. A. Regier (Eds.), *Psychiatric disorders in America: The epidemiologic catchment area study* (pp. 116–154). New York, NY: Free Press.

Banerjee, S., Clancy, C., & Crome, I. (2002). Co-existing problems of mental disorder and substance misuse (dual diagnosis): An information manual. Retrieved from http://www.rcpsych.ac.uk

Berman, S., & Noble, E. P. (1993). Childhood antecedents of substance misuse. *Current Opinion in Psychiatry*, *6*(3), 382–387. doi:10.1097/00001504-199306000-00012

Parrino, M. W., Severtson, S. G., Bucher-Bartelson, B., & Green J. L. Trends in opioid analgesic abuse and mortality in the United States. *The New England Journal of Medicine*, *372*(3), 241–248.

References

Dart, R. C., Surratt, H. L., Cicero, T. J., Parrino, M. W., Severtson, S. G., Bucher-Bartelson, B., & Green, J. L. (2015). Trends in opioid analgesic abuse and mortality in the United States. *New England Journal of Medicine*, *372*(3), 241–248.

Hedden, S. L., Kennet, J., Lipari, R., Medley, G., & Tice, P. (2014). SAMSHA Center for Behavioral Health Statistics and Quality. (2015). *Behavioral health trends in the United States: Results from the 2014 Nation Survey on Drug Use and Health* (HHS Publication No. SMA 15-4927, NSDUH Series H-50). Retrieved from http://www.samhsa.gov/data/sites/default/les/NSDUH-FRR1-2014/NSDUH-FRR1-2014.pdf

Substance Abuse and Mental Health Services Administration. (2014). Results from the 2013 National Survey on Drug Use and Health: Mental health findings. Retrieved from http://www.samhsa.gov/data/sites/default/files/NSDUHmhfr2013/NSDUHmhfr2013.htm

United States Department of Health and Human Services. (2015). The opioid epidemic: By the numbers. Retrieved from https://www.hhs.gov/sites/default/files/Factsheet-opioids-061516.pdf

United States Department of Health & Human Services. (2016). The opioid epidemic by the numbers. Retrieved from https://www.hhs.gov/sites/default/files/Factsheet-opioids-061516.pdf

Volkow, B. (2014). Prescription opioid and heroin abuse. Retrieved from https://www.drugabuse.gov/about-nida/legislative-activities/testimony-to-congress/2016/prescription-opioid-heroin-abuse#5

Website Resources

Evidence-based practice & toolkits: Implementation of integrated dual diagnosis treatment (IDDT): http://slideplayer.com/slide/6637092

The opioid epidemic: HHS: www.hhs.gov/sites/default/files/Factsheet-opioids-061516.pdf

Screening for and assessment of co-occurring substance use and mental health disorders by alcohol and other drug and mental health services (Victorian Dual Diagnosis Initiative) by G. Croton (2007): www.nada.org.au/media/14706/vddi_screening.pdf

U.S. Department of Health & Human Services (HHS): www.hhs.gov/opioids/about-the-epidemic

16

Challenges in Treating Substance Use Disorders and Dual Diagnosis

In this chapter, you will learn:

- How pain, mental illness, and substance use disorders (SUDs) overlap
- Nursing's position statement on pain management for patients with SUDs
- Special considerations when assessing and managing pain in patients with mental illness and dual diagnosis
- Issues related to addictive disorders in health care professionals
- What recovery comprises
- Alternative therapies for managing pain
- Important nursing considerations regarding use of pain medications in patients with mental illness and SUDs

The American Academy of Pain Medicine (n.d.), in the *AAPM Facts and Figures on Pain,* notes that 26% of Americans older than 20 years of age (76.2 million people) have some type of pain condition, whether acute or chronic. The four most common types of reported pain are back pain, migraine, and neck and facial ache or pain, with back pain the most common disability in the United States (Centers for Disease Control and Prevention, 2010). About 15% to 25% of Americans report living with chronic pain, and the presence of pain increases the likelihood of mental illness, addiction, and suicide (Ilgen et al., 2013; Means-Christensen, Roy-Byme, Sherbourne, Craske, & Stein, 2008). Pain management in the United States has a cost that is higher than treating cardiovascular disease, cancer, and accidental injuries (Steiner, 2014).

The primary medications prescribed for pain management are opiates. Although these narcotics are effective in reducing pain, they affect the patient's ability to function in daily life and should not, except in cases of terminal illness, be used as a long-term solution. As discussed in Chapter 15, extended use of narcotics can lead to tolerance, requiring higher doses and more frequent usage to obtain the same results.

This chapter highlights challenges in working with patients who, along with mental illness or dual diagnosis, also require management of chronic or acute pain needs. Also included are statistics related to SUDs among health professionals and strategies that nurses can employ to support anyone with an SUD or psychiatric disorder in moving toward recovery.

PAIN, MENTAL ILLNESS, AND SUDs

As Von Korff et al. (2005) note, pain is a comorbid condition for those with SUDs, most commonly alcohol use. Overall, 10% of patients in primary care environments complaining of noncancer-related pain have a concurrent SUD, while those in specialty areas have a 10% to 30% rate (Morasco, Duckart, & Dobscha, 2011). Conversely, almost half of all patients in treatment for SUDs report having pain with rates higher when the dependency being treated is opioid addiction (Potter, Shiffman, & Weiss, 2008). When a patient has a concurrent SUD and pain diagnosis, the prognosis is poor, as abstinence from the substance often fuels the pain, and suboptimal treatment of the pain can undermine abstinence. It is important to clarify that when a patient with a prescription for a drug *is taking it as directed by a medical professional*, the continued use of the medication does not constitute an SUD.

Patients who have chronic medical conditions often also experience depression. Dysphoria is commonly seen in those being treated for cancer, heart disease, metabolic diseases, epilepsy, vascular diseases, neurological disorders, and connective tissue conditions. The National Institute of Mental Health identifies chronic disease as a risk factor for depression, and depression and other mental illnesses as risk factors for developing chronic diseases.

As health professionals, we need to understand and recognize the need for all the patient's presenting symptoms to be addressed. The best method for working with these complex patient issues is to clearly identify the individual's presenting problems, symptoms, and health needs and then prioritize the care based on the evidence. Multiple methods, outside of use of opiates, are available to health professionals to treat pain. Different psychiatric disorders require specialized interventions, many of which do not interfere with providing effective pain management. Although it is true that the recent increased prescription rate of opioids has been matched with the increased level of opioid drug abuse and overdoses, not all who take opioid medications for pain will progress to abuse of the medications. Lastly, the existence of an acute or chronic condition that is causing pain and suffering for a patient should be explored and treated by the medical team on its own merits with evidence-based methods.

NURSING'S POSITION STATEMENT ON PAIN MANAGEMENT FOR PATIENTS WITH SUDs

The American Society for Pain Management Nursing (ASPMN) and the International Nurses Society on Addictions (IntNSA) hold the position that patients with substance use disorders and pain have the right to be treated with dignity, respect, and the same quality of pain assessment and management as all other patients. Safe and effective care of patients with substance use disorders includes maintaining a balance between the provision of pain relief, monitoring for appropriate use of prescribed medications and other substances, and recommendations for viable treatment alternatives. Nurses are well positioned and obligated to advocate for pain management across all treatment settings for patients at various points along a continuum of substance use (Oliver et al., 2012).

Various conceptual models of addiction and treatment have directed nursing actions over the years. They include:

- The *moral and criminal model*, in which the person with the addiction disorder is judged to be morally flawed.
- The *disease model*, in which the disorder is identified as a neurological, dopaminergic pathway disorder affecting impulse and executive decision making.

- The *bio-psycho-social-spiritual* model, which incorporates the interaction of multiple systems, internal and external, in affecting the individual's sense of self.
- The *12-step model*, in which the individual identifies the foundational spiritual crisis and, after professing powerlessness over the behavior, finds spiritual strength to change behaviors (Oliver et al., 2012).

As these models make clear, there are multiple approaches to providing care for the person with a substance disorder who requires pain management. One approach, the moral and criminal model, although accepted by some institutions, predisposes the patient to biased care. The other three models take into consideration the complicated challenges of treating the patient with a dual diagnosis. Regardless of the model used, the nurse is obligated to provide the best patient care to the patient with pain and a coexisting SUD. Each nurse, whether practicing at the level of a staff RN or a practitioner/prescriber, must maintain the objectivity required to treat the whole person, not the diagnosis. These patients often present nurses with a real practice challenge. They demand that we listen carefully, assess needs with the patient's story in mind, and keep any preexisting biases or personal experiences out of our judgment. Recommendations on how to accomplish this in the clinical setting can be found in Table 16.1.

ADDICTIVE DISORDERS IN HEALTH CARE PROFESSIONALS

Addiction is a problem that affects health care professionals along with the general public. It is estimated that one in 10 physicians has a drug or alcohol use disorder, or both (Merlo, Singhakant, Cummings, & Cottle, 2013). Ten percent to 15% of nurses are believed to have an addictive disorder (Thomas & Siela, 2011). Nurses have not been found to misuse alcohol or illicit drugs more than people in other professions. However, 10% of nurses have been identified as having a drinking problem, which translates into 2.2 million nurses. Additionally, use of prescription drugs by nurses is higher than in the general public, with a higher prevalence among critical care nurses and emergency department nurses. Some of the factors that are seen as increasing the likelihood of drug use among physicians and nurses include high stress, easy access, and emotional pain. Working alongside a colleague who is abusing drugs or alcohol can put your patient's life and your professional future in jeopardy.

Table 16.1

Recommendations for Nurses, Prescribers, and Institutions to Optimize the Care of Patients With Concomitant Pain and SUDs

Care provider or setting	Actions
Nursing Practice	■ Stay abreast of current knowledge in the evolving fields of pain management and SUDs. ■ Advocate for best practices and provide nonbiased, evidence-based care. ■ Contribute through research, education, and clinical practice to the development of holistic nursing models.
Prescriber/Provider Practice	■ Remain up to date with an understanding of pain management and SUDs. ■ Demonstrate and model best practices. ■ Use safe prescribing protocols with options for individualization if needed. ■ Refer for appropriate specialty care. ■ Advocate as needed for this marginalized population.
Institution	■ Engage key stakeholders in the establishment of policies or protocols to ensure that appropriate expertise, therapies, and resources are available. ■ Convene clinical practice committees charged with reviewing the practice of nurses, pharmacists, physicians, and any provider caring for patients with persistent pain or SUDs. Call on pharmacy and therapeutic committees to ensure optimal access to care. ■ Institute quality assurance processes to monitor appropriateness and efficacy of care.

SUD, substance use disorder.

Source: Oliver et al. (2012).

The National Council of State Boards of Nursing has produced a resource manual and guidelines for alternative and disciplinary monitoring programs. A resource link to this publication is found in the website references at the end of the chapter. Health care providers can use prescription drugs, illegally obtain prescription drugs and street drugs, as well as abuse alcohol. Sometimes an exposure to a traumatic event can trigger a response of self-medication. It is not always easy to identify the medical professional with a drug or alcohol problem, and compulsive use of substances is not a choice that someone makes. Addiction is a serious disease. Addiction in nurses, physicians, and other health care providers can cause increased patient morbidity and mortality, and put other professional colleagues' licenses at risk. If you see something, say something. Table 16.2 is a useful checklist for identifying signs and symptoms of abuse in a health care provider.

WHAT IS RECOVERY?

"Recovery" is a broad term that encompasses individuals who are receiving treatment for mental disorders or SUDs. It reflects the current, best evidence, on the part of the Substance Abuse and Mental Health Services Administration (SAMHSA) and the Institute of Medicine (IOM), that anyone who works at managing his or her mental illness or SUD can recover.

Table 16.2

Checklist of Symptoms of the Drug-Addicted Nurse

1. Extreme and rapid mood swings: irritable with patients, then calm after taking drugs
2. Suspicious behavior concerning controlled drugs:
   - Consistently signs out more controlled drugs than anyone else
   - Frequently breaks or spills drugs
   - Purposely waits until alone to open narcotics cabinet
   - Consistently volunteers to be med nurse
   - Disappears into bathroom directly after being in narcotics cabinet
   - Vials appear altered
   - Incorrect narcotic count
   - Discrepancies between patients' reports and other patient's reports on effective medications, etc.
   - Patient complains that pain medication dispensed by the nurse are ineffective
   - Defensive when asked about medication errors
3. Illogical or sloppy charting
4. Frequently absent from unit
5. Comes to work early and stays late for no reason; hangs around
6. Lavishly uses sick leave

Source: Ohio Board of Nursing (1999).

Fast Facts in the Spotlight

SAMHSA's Definition of Recovery: Recovery is seen as a change process helping people achieve better health and well-being. SAMHSA is continually updating its definition as our understanding of the importance of a holistic approach to recovery emerges. Through recovery people can engage in self-directed behaviors, allowing them to reach their fullest potential. The process of recovery supports individuals to improve their physical and emotional health and wellness, live self-directed lives, and strive to reach their full potential. There are many pathways to recovery, including the need for understanding the importance of culture, community, hope, and respect. Access to clinical treatments and support services that are evidence based for all persons, is the foundation of SAMHSA's definition of recovery (SAMHSA, 2016).

The four dimensions identified by SAMHSA that support recovery are:

1. Health—Defined as a person's ability to overcome or manage his or her disease to the extent that the individual is able to make positive outcome choices supportive of emotional and physical health.
2. Home—For recovery, a person needs to have a place in which to reside that is safe and stable.
3. Purpose—Getting involved in activities that are meaningful and are attended on a regular basis, allowing the individual to contribute to the greater society.
4. Community—The development of relationships that convey the belief that each person, with support, can overcome his or her challenges and create a meaningful, fulfilling life.

Programs that have been developed to support recovery seek to increase the resilience of the person by teaching strategies to help him or her cope with challenges and prepare for setbacks. The importance of social networks and individual relationships is paramount, and often it is the therapeutic relationship with a nurse, during a brief encounter, that can start a patient thinking about recovery.

Recovery Programs

SAMHSA, the Institute of Medicine, and the Surgeon General of the United States support recovery programs for all people dealing with substance use and mental health disorders. To this end, Recovery to Practice programs have been developed by different professional groups and are available through SAMHSA. A nurse-focused, recovery-oriented program developed by the American Psychiatric Nurses Association (APNA, 2015) provides evidence-based strategies in an easy-to-follow curriculum that increases nursing knowledge for care that facilitates patient recovery. This is a six-module course that, in alignment with the SAMHSA initiative, introduces recovery principles, increases awareness of mental health recovery, and provides the foundation to implement a Recovery to Practice program. The APNA program (R2P) can be obtained through contact with APNA (2017).

Recovery programs address multiple populations from school-aged children to geriatric adults. All Recovery to Practice programs, however, have one thing in common: they all must meet specific SAMHSA qualifications. They must be evidence based, must respect and respond to diverse cultural and linguistic needs of the populations they serve, must address diversity for service delivery, and must include a focus on health disparity reduction related to both access to services and outcome measures. The programs seek to reduce social isolation, decrease the stigma of mental illness and SUDs, and build a better, measurable recovery that improves the quality of life it serves.

ALTERNATIVE MEASURES FOR PAIN MANAGEMENT

The Joint Commission on Accreditation of Healthcare Organizations (JCAHO) and the World Health Organization (WHO) have provided a stepladder approach to treating pain. There are three approaches to pain mitigation, depending upon whether the presenting pain is acute, chronic, or end of life. In some cases, use of "around-the-clock" standing orders for pain control provides higher levels of pain management, even when the drug of choice is an opioid, as the purpose is pain relief. The WHO's stepladder approach to pain management for prescribers can be found online (Prater, Zylstra, & Miller, 2002).

Unfortunately, patients with SUDs are less likely than those in the general population to experience adequate pain treatment. The problem the prescriber faces is that if the pain is not adequately treated, the patient will seek alternative drugs to self-medicate and is more likely to experience a full relapse. All medical professionals should be working to provide adequate pain relief for the patient experiencing pain. The patient, not the provider, is the best judge of the level of pain and should be allowed to provide information (either by a chart or scale) to establish level of pain.

Pain that presents as part of a medical emergency must be treated as the medical emergency and adequately controlled as inadequate medication can increase the pain experience and the degree of difficulty in treating it. Some patients might present with a phenomenon of *pseudoaddiction,* in which their behaviors mimic active addictive behaviors, usually due to prior experiences with inadequate pain medication. These patients often ask for far more medication than appears necessary for the proportion of pain displayed, and they may hoard the pain medications. Careful development of the therapeutic alliance and constructing a respectful environment in which the patient's voice can be heard may reduce the occurrence of this phenomenon.

Depending on the origin of the pain, opioids may not be the first line of medication considered for treatment. For example, if the presenting problem is bone pain, the use of nonsteroidal anti-inflammatory agents could be more appropriate. When end-of-life issues are related to pain management, the prescriber should not be concerned primarily with the addictive disorder, but rather with adequate pain management and the collaboration to achieve it that will occur between the patient and prescriber.

Fast Facts in the Spotlight

Did you know that atypical antipsychotic, antidepressants, and anti-seizure medications are sometimes used to decrease pain in patients with chronic pain problems? When taking the history, and learning the medications your patient is taking, it is important to ask *why* the patient is taking the medication—not just what medication is being taken. Use of certain drugs can precipitate acute withdrawal if the patient is opioid dependent.

ALTERNATIVE THERAPIES FOR MANAGING PAIN

Therapeutic interventions that are used instead of, or in conjunction with, pain medications include some of the techniques of alternative and complementary medicine. These approaches involve multiple disciplines from acupuncture to chiropractic medicine and can include various forms of healing touch, meditation, yoga, aromatherapy, biofeedback, and herbal medications. Nurses should be familiar with the approaches that are commonly integrated within the health care setting.

Acupuncture

In this traditional Chinese medical approach, trained acupuncture practitioners use thin needles to stimulate specific energy points on the body. The most common use of acupuncture is pain management, including chronic pain management, migraines, osteoarthritis, and low back pain. Use of nonsterile needles can result in complications from this approach.

Healing Touch, Therapeutic Touch, and Reiki

Healing Touch

Healing Touch, a nursing intervention that involves laying of hands, was developed in 1989 by Janet Mentgen and is endorsed by the American Holistic Nurses Association. Practitioners use several techniques, including chakra, magnetic fields, chelation, and lymphatic release, to increase physical and emotional health. Practitioners receive certification in a five-level process through Healing Touch International.

Therapeutic Touch

Therapeutic Touch, considered another laying of hands technique, was developed in the 1970s by Dolores Kreiger, a nurse, and Dora Kunz, a healer. The underlying theory posits that practitioners are able to direct a universal energy field toward physical and emotional healing. The steps used by therapeutic touch practitioners are assessment, clearing, energy balancing, repatterning of energy, and closure of field.

Reiki

Reiki is an ancient Japanese technique that uses laying of hands to increase relaxation and decrease stress. It is based on the belief that the practitioner can channel universal life-force energy to the patient, promoting healing. There are three levels of certification for Reiki practitioners.

Meditation and Other Mind–Body Therapies

Meditation

"Meditation" is a general term used to describe techniques for increasing "mindfulness" through quiet reflection and contemplation. There are many different forms of meditation practice, from personal mindfulness, during which a person may sit and observe the world, withholding all judgment, to transcendental meditation, which is a structured meditation practice. Some meditation includes the practice of yoga, which includes body postures and breath control in addition to reflection, while others use the chakra energy centers of the body for the focus of the thoughtful contemplation. A short explanation of 11 different types of meditations can be found online at mindful minutes.com/meditation-styles-techniques-explained.

Mind–Body Therapies

Mind–body therapies are interventions that include the contemplative aspect of meditation with a body-centered action. These approaches include relaxation interventions, directed/positive imagery exercises, cognitive behavioral therapy (CBT), and sensorimotor psychotherapy. Some of these (e.g., relaxation and imagery) can be done by the patient alone while others (e.g., CBT and sensorimotor psychotherapy) need to be done in collaboration with a trained therapist.

NURSING CONSIDERATIONS WHEN PROVIDING PAIN MANAGEMENT TO PATIENTS USING PSYCHOTROPIC MEDICATIONS

When taking the history from the patient or patient's family, ask clear questions that can be delivered without judgment. For example, rather than asking, "You don't take any illicit drugs, do you?" you might say, "Tell me about any medicine you have taken in the past week, for your pain and for any other reason. Please include both prescription and nonprescription, over-the-counter medications, herbs, and anything a friend might have provided to you to help with the pain. Let me know of any medication that you might have taken as a pill, a drink, smoked, or injected." If you find that your patient is taking two or more prescribed medications, consult with your pharmacist or a pocket or web-based pharmacology reference (e.g., www.epocrates.com) for any known drug-to-drug interaction.

Fast Facts in the Spotlight

In all cases, it is especially important to get a full list of the medications (prescribed, illicitly used prescription drugs, over-the-counter drugs, herbs, and illicit drugs) from all patients. Drug–drug reactions, even when the medications are delivered in the hospital, can cause respiratory depression or acute withdrawal and are life-threatening emergencies (SAMHSA, 2016).

Questions to Ask

Some nursing questions to pose to your patients with chronic pain to evaluate whether their use of medications has gone from therapeutic to misuse of substance in the self-treatment of pain include the following:

- Are you taking pain medication that belongs to another person for relief?
- Do you go to different doctors to get more prescriptions for pain medication?
- Are you taking the medications for pain differently than the way they have been prescribed?
- Do you ever use your pain medication when you do not have pain?

SPOTLIGHT ON THE UNIT: APPLYING KNOWLEDGE TO PRACTICE—MEDICATION DILEMMAS

An 18-year-old woman comes to the minute clinic to see the nurse. She explains that she took a pregnancy test, which showed she is pregnant. She has been using oxycodone recreationally for 5 weeks, three times a day (sometimes more) in addition to bupropion HCl XL, 150 mg/day PO, which she has taken for 3 years for depression and attention deficit disorder. She tells you that she wants to keep the baby and doesn't want to take the oxycodone anymore, so she got some buprenorphine pills from a friend. She

(continued)

wants to take these because her friend told her they would help her stop being addicted to the oxycodone.

- What can you advise her?
- To whom should you refer her?
- Is this an emergency?
- What are your priorities?

TAKE-AWAY

Pain management is a complex issue that is central to the delivery of safe, effective patient care, even without the added complications of mental illness or SUDs. The person who presents with pain as the chief complaint requires attention to evaluate and address the pain. Often the co-occurrence of a mental illness or SUD can impact the health care practitioner's judgment, switching the need from pain relief to dealing with the chronic disease of mental illness first. It is important to reflect on the factors that can interrupt best practice, while keeping the needs of the patient in the forefront of care delivery.

Further Reading

American Psychiatric Association. (2013). *Diagnostic and statistical manual of mental disorders* (5th ed.). Arlington, VA: American Psychiatric Publishing.

Anthony, J. C., & Helzer, J. E. (1991). Syndromes of drug abuse and dependence. In L. N. Robins & D. A. Regier (Eds.), *Psychiatric disorders in America: The epidemiologic catchment area study* (pp. 116–154). New York, NY: Free Press.

Banerjee, S., Clancy, C., & Crome, I. (2002). Co-existing problems of mental disorder and substance misuse (dual diagnosis): An information manual. Retrieved from http://www.rcpsych.ac.uk

Dart, R. C., Surratt, H. L., Cicero, T. J., Parrino, M. W., Severtson, G., Bucher-Bartelson, B., & Green, J. L. (2015). Trends in opioid analgesic abuse and mortality in the United States. *New England Journal of Medicine, 372*(3), 241–248. doi: 10.1056/NEJMsa1406143

National Institute on Drug Abuse. (2014, January 1). Principles of adolescent substance use disorder: A research-based guide. Retrieved from www.drugabuse.gov/publications/principles-adolescent-substance-use-disorder-treatment-research-based-guide/introduction

Ohio Board of Nursing. (1999). Signs and symptoms of the alcoholic nurse. Retrieved from https://www.ahcmedia.com/articles/41166-signs-and-symptoms-of-the-alcoholic-nurse

Stahl, S., & Grady. M. (2012). *Stahl's illustrated substance use and impulsive disorders.* Cambridge, UK: Cambridge University Press.

Substance Abuse and Mental Health Services Administration. (2012). SAMHSA's working definition of recovery updated. Retrieved from https://blog.samhsa.gov/2012/03/23/defintion-of-recovery-updated/#.WRjL1BPyvVo

Substance Abuse and Mental Health Services Administration. (2015). Recovery and recovery support. Retrieved from http://www.samhsa.gov/recovery

Trinkoff, A., & Storr C. (1998). Substance use among nurses: Differences between specialties. *American Journal of Public Health, 88,* 581–585.

Vickers, A. J., & Linde, K. (2014). Acupuncture for chronic pain. *Journal of the American Medical Association, 311*(9), 955–956.

References

American Academy of Pain Medicine. (n.d.) Facts and figures on pain. Retrieved from http://www.painmed.org/files/facts-and-figures-on-pain.pdf

American Psychiatric Nurses Association. (2015). APNA recovery to practice program. Retrieved from http://www.apna.org/i4a/pages/index.cfm?pageID=5296

Centers for Disease Control and Prevention. (2010, December). QuickStats: Percentage of adults who had migraines or severe headaches, pain in the neck, lower back, or face/jaw, by sex—National Health Interview Survey, 2009. *Morbidity and Mortality Weekly Report, 59*(47), 1557. Retrieved from https://www.cdc.gov/mmwr/preview/mmwrhtml/mm5947a6.htm

Ilgen, M., Kleinberg, F., Ignacio, R., Bohnert, A. S., Valenstein, M., McCarthy, J. F., . . . Katz, I. R. (2013). Noncancer pain conditions and risk of suicide. *Journal of the American Medical Association Psychiatry, 70*(7), 692–697.

Means-Christensen, A. J., Roy-Byme, P. P., Sherbourne, C. D., Craske, M. G., & Stein, M. B. (2008). Relationships among pain, anxiety, and depression in primary care. *Depression and Anxiety, 25*(7), 593–600.

Merlo, L., Singhakant, S., Cummings, S., & Cottler, L. (2013). Reasons for misuse of prescription medication among physicians undergoing monitoring by a physician health program. *Journal of Addiction Medicine, 7*(5), 349–353.

Morasco, B. J., Duckart, J. P., & Dobscha, S. K. (2011). Adherence to clinical guidelines for opioid therapy for chronic pain in patients with substance use disorder. *Journal of General Internal Medicine, 26*(9), 965–971.

Ohio Board of Nursing. (1999). Signs and symptoms of the drug-addicted nurse. Retrieved from https://www.ahcmedia.com/articles/41170-signs-and-symptoms-of-the-drug-addicted-nurse

Oliver, J., Coggins, C., Compton, P., Hagan, S., Matteliano, D., Stanton, M., . . . Turner, H. (2012). American Society for Pain Management Nursing Position Statement: Pain management in patients with substance use disorders. *Pain Management Nursing: Official Journal of the American Society of Pain Management Nurses, 13*(3), 169–183. doi:10.1016/j.pmn .2012.07.001

Potter, J. S., Shiffman, S. J., & Weiss, R. D. (2008). Chronic pain severity in opioid-dependent patients. *American Journal of Drug and Alcohol Abuse, 34*(1), 101–107.

Prater, C. D., Zylstra, R. G., & Miller, K. E. (2002). Successful pain management for the recovering addicted patient. *Primary Care Companion to the Journal of Clinical Psychiatry, 4*(4), 125–131. Retrieved from https://www .ncbi.nlm.nih.gov/pmc/articles/PMC315480/table/i1523-5998-004-04 -0125-t01

Steiner, B. (2014, April). Treating chronic pain with meditation. *The Atlantic Magazine.* Retrieved from https://www.theatlantic.com/health/archive/ 2014/04/treating-chronic-pain-with-meditation/284182

Substance Abuse and Mental Health Services Administration. (2016). SAMHSA's working definition of recovery: 10 guiding principles of recovery. Retrieved from https://store.samhsa.gov/shin/content/PEP12 -RECDEF/PEP12-RECDEF.pdf

Thomas, C., & Siela, D. (2011). The impaired nurse: Would you know what to do if you suspected substance abuse? *American Nurse Today, 6*(8). Retrieved from https://www.americannursetoday.com/the-impaired-nurse -would-you-know-what-to-do-if-you-suspected-substance-abuse

Von Korff, M., Crane, P., Lane, M., Miglioretti, D. L., Simon, G., Saunders, K., . . . Kessler R. (2005). Chronic spinal pain and physical–mental comorbidity in the United States: Results from the National Comorbidity Survey replication. *Pain, 113*, 331–339.

V

Psychiatric/Mental Health Issues: Clinical Setting Challenges

17

Treating the Mentally Ill Outside the Psychiatric Unit: A Review

In this chapter, you will learn:

- About challenges and strategies when caring for psychiatric patients in the following settings:
    - Criminal justice system
    - Emergency department or urgi-centers
    - Obstetric, labor, delivery, and newborn units
    - Medical–surgical units
    - Intensive care units (ICU, MICU, SICU, PACU)
    - School health settings
- Nursing strategies for working with mentally ill patients in varied settings

Patients with psychiatric disorders are scattered throughout hospital units, receiving treatment for other medical issues and emergencies in addition to the required specialized treatment of their psychiatric diagnoses. A decline in the number of inpatient beds for psychiatric patients is reflected in the increasing numbers of these patients being seen in primary care environments, being referred to specialty out-patient programs, utilizing community and self-help organizations, and entering the criminal justice system.

Fast Facts in the Spotlight

There is an acute shortage of psychiatric inpatient beds in the United States. The Treatment Advocacy Center reports that the number of beds in the past 50 years has decreased by 95%. At the same time, the number of mentally ill patients continues to rise, with one in four Americans experiencing some kind of mental illness.

Providing safe, effective, evidence-based care is the foundation of all nursing interventions. The privilege of nursing is that we are often the first human hand, and the last one, to touch a life. We intervene to facilitate healing in *all* people who seek medical help. As nurses, we are among the most highly trusted professionals because of our ability to form meaningful alliances with our patients—relationships that have positive effects on their ability to heal. Our profession prides itself on the ability to exhibit compassion that is coupled with clinical competence, advocacy that is connected to accessibility, evidence-based care that also reflects genuine empathy, and interventions that are ethically sound.

Patients who receive a psychiatric diagnosis require good nursing care in order to obtain relief and move toward or remain in recovery. The more you know about your patients, and the better versed you are about psychiatric diseases, the better your nursing care will be. The following strategies can help ensure excellent caregiving regardless of unit or diagnosis.

- *Knowledge:* Be aware of what you know and what you need to know. Then get the factual, evidence-based answers to the questions you need to know.
- *Safety:* Create a safe environment. Evaluate the environment for safety issues that could be present for the patient, staff, or visitors. Identify anything that could be unsafe and, where possible, mitigate the hazard. Reduce stimuli where possible and provide support and understanding to reduce stress and anxiety responses from the patient and the patient's family. Follow policies and guidelines for use of restraints (physical and chemical).
- *Mindfulness*: Be aware of what you feel and think, and realize that thoughts and feelings can alter behaviors. Be honest in your

self-inventory and seek help if your thoughts, beliefs, fears, or emotional reactions are interfering with your ability to provide good, safe, effective nursing care.

■ *Availability:* Be present for the patient. Listen to the patient and collaborate as part of the patient's team. There is no "fix" for mental illness. It is a chronic, usually progressive disease to which patients adapt. Work with the patient to achieve the best outcome. Use simple, directive "I" statements; for example, "I am going to take your temperature; I need you to open your mouth for me." Provide the patient enough time to listen, process, and respond to the command.

■ *Support and referrals:* Identify when you need to have more support in order to gather information (family), provide safe care (staff), restrain (staff, police, response team), or provide specific psychiatric interventions (psychiatric consult). Use toolkits and surveys, many of which are available online, to help assess needs (e.g., crosscutting symptoms measurement tools, available at www.psychiatry.org/psychiatrists/practice/dsm/dsm-5/online-assessment-measures).

SPECIFIC CHALLENGES IN SPECIALTY UNITS AND WORKPLACES

Criminal Justice System (Jails and Prisons)

Prisoners with psychiatric disorders in these settings:

■ Have longer lengths of stay due to homelessness, rule breaking, and no reduction of prison time
■ Cause behavioral problems for other inmates
■ Are more likely to be beaten or raped during incarceration
■ Have symptom exacerbation during prison terms if not treated
■ Spend more time in isolation/solitary confinement
■ Are more likely to become recidivists (revolving door return to prison)
■ Have higher rates of suicide

Emergency Departments and Urgi-Centers

Patients with psychiatric disorders in these settings:

■ Are more likely to have longer lengths of stay due to the low number of psychiatric beds for referral

- Face more fear and bias from staff and attending health care professionals due to lack of psychiatric specialists
- Require a safe space, for both the patient and staff
- Will require more staff for 1:1 observations
- Have a higher risk for unpredictable behaviors, including violence
- Have complex problem presentations, often including substance use disorders and drug-seeking behaviors
- Should be assessed for suicide risk and monitored if found at risk using the following questions:
  - Do you have any thoughts of killing yourself? (Intention)
  - Do you have a plan? (Plan)
  - Are you able to carry out your plan? (Ability)

Obstetrics, Labor, Delivery, and Newborn Units

Patients with psychiatric disorders who are pregnant or have just delivered present challenges specific to the obstetric/postpartum unit. It is especially important to recognize when a patient expresses extreme sadness or anxiety during the labor and immediate postpartum period. Patients with preexisting depression or a history of postpartum depression are at a higher risk for having a depressive disorder again. Patients in these settings:

- Are at increased risk of perinatal and postpartum depression
- May have other psychosocial difficulties, including homelessness, divorce, joblessness, family history of abuse, and lack of health insurance
- May have a psychiatric illness that is only now presenting due to the increased stress and hormonal changes of pregnancy
- Have a higher likelihood of self-care deficits
- Face stigma related to taking psychiatric medications during pregnancy
- May have more difficulties in breastfeeding and fulfilling other parenting responsibilities

Medical–Surgical Units

Many patients who take psychotropic drugs for extended periods develop metabolic syndrome, as well as other ailments consistent with normal aging. Nurses frequently encounter these patients on the medical–surgical unit. Patients in these settings:

- Have more dependency issues, requiring the nurse to spend more time with them (or to assign someone to sit with them for observation)
- Are more likely to behave unpredictably
- May engage in "cheeking" (placing medication into the cheek rather than swallowing it)
- Are more likely to refuse treatment or routine testing

Intensive Care Units (ICU, MICU, SICU, PACU)

Patients with psychiatric disorders in these settings:

- May experience acute fear responses and require increased sedation
- Are more likely to remove intravenous lines and electronic monitoring devices
- Require 1:1 surveillance

In addition to encountering patients in the ICU who have a preexisting psychiatric diagnosis, nurses may care for patients who develop psychotic responses as a result of a prolonged stay in the ICU (referred to as "ICU psychosis"). Depression is often a secondary diagnosis that patients experience after an ICU experience.

Pediatrics and School Health Environments

Children are often "invisible" psychiatric patients, with many learning at very young ages how to hide their emotional pain from family and other adults. The somatic complaints that indicate an emotional storm can be confirmed by the child, or dispelled by the parents. The school nurse and the pediatric nurse often provide children with the first trustable grownup with whom they can share their stories. It is a difficult position to occupy, as nurses must be ready to report any incidence—or suspicion—of child abuse when findings so indicate.

School or pediatric nurses who provide care to children with psychiatric disorders may observe the following signs and symptoms:

- Frequent visits for nonspecific complaints
- Increased impulsivity
- Hopelessness, lack of joy
- Lack of energy, sleep disturbances
- Sudden weight gain or loss

- Increased use of substances
- Unexplained and denied injuries (burning, scratching, picking)

Nursing interventions in these settings focus on assessing the child's risk for self-injury and suicide, creating a safe space, and referral to a pediatric mental health specialist.

STRATEGIES FOR WORKING WITH ALL PATIENTS, AND ESPECIALLY THOSE WITH MENTAL ILLNESS

Assess the Patient Thoroughly

Conduct the normal head-to-toe evaluation that you would perform for all patients. Patients with a psychiatric problem may not always tell you about it when seeking care for a different, medical problem or from another medical provider. Often the experience of stigma at the hands of other health professionals makes patients very worried about exposing their full mental health history.

Maintain a Safe Environment

Pay attention to what you are hearing, seeing, and learning from the patient. Ask direct questions when you feel a patient may have a possible psychiatric problem that could result in harm to self or others. Examples include:

- Do you want to kill yourself? (Refer to suicide risk questions, earlier.)
- Are you hearing voices that no one else can hear?
- Do you have any thoughts about hurting anyone? Yourself or anyone else?

Listen respectfully to the response, and determine what actions are necessary. In the case of patients with psychotic symptoms who report "hearing voices," are these command voices that might tell them to hurt themselves or someone else? Keep the patient, yourself, and others in the environment safe. Refer the patient to a psychiatric/mental health specialist if one is available.

Evaluate Level of Emotional Distress (The Patient's and Yours!)

In stress-filled environments everyone can act on edge, somewhat uncooperative, and simply "not like one's normal self." Stressful environments present an especially difficult challenge for the mentally ill. Once the patient's defense mechanisms are activated, he or she might respond with fight, flight, freeze, or submit behaviors. These behaviors provide insight into the patient's inability to engage the executive level of thinking to persevere through the situation. Patients with a history of trauma may have their memories rekindled, and they might re-experience their trauma, making treatment more challenging.

- *Fight (i.e., Violence):* A fearful patient can respond to demands with aggression if he or she feels threatened. It is important to observe for the first signs of agitation with a patient and work to de-escalate the problem.
- *Flight:* The patient preparing to flee may appear to be in a hyper-aroused state, intensely watching all who enter and leave the room, and looking at all the exits. Such patients may ask a flurry of questions related to what might happen next, but, when left alone, head for the nearest exit.
- *Freeze:* The patient who freezes typically displays prodromal symptoms of trauma, such as skin tingling, numbing, or emotional withdrawal. The freezing might take on a sense of purposeful mutism, if the provider is not aware that the patient has become emotionally overwhelmed.
- *Submit:* The patient who submits as a fear response will tell you whatever it is that he or she believes you expect as the desired response. This trauma response is often misinterpreted as cooperation, but it involves lack of collaboration on the part of the patient. The clinical presentation is that of a patient who does what is asked, but who is emotionally not present.

When such behaviors occur, it is important that the nurse and the health care team respond in a way that restores calm and safety to the environment.

Be Aware of Passive-Aggressive Responses

Passive-aggressive behavior is demonstrated by patients who state a willingness to follow the requested nursing demands but specifically go against the requested behaviors. This response is sometimes interpreted by health care providers as being stubborn, willful, or negative. Staff who react to this kind of behavior with increased agitation will only escalate the instability of the environment. Patients, however, are not the only people who engage in passive-aggressive behaviors. Health professionals who use passive-aggressive strategies in their personal lives might also find themselves engaging in this behavior on the unit. Self-awareness is imperative when working with the mentally ill.

Be Aware of Professionals' Engagement in Microaggression With Mentally Ill Patients

Microaggression is very similar to passive-aggression, but it is conducted on a more subtle level and often reflects a belief that is so ingrained in the aggressor that it is not even a conscious attack. Individuals with mental illness, however, are very sensitive to the reactions of others toward their diagnosis. This type of aggression includes having a dismissive attitude toward the complaints or symptoms of the patient, or possibly minimizing the person's experiences because the patient "doesn't seem that crazy."

Another type of microaggressive behavior occurs when the nurse "symptomizes" the patient, interpreting the patient's normal responses as a suspicious symptom of the disorder. It is sometimes difficult for a nurse who is not a psychiatric specialist to find the comfort zone between minimizing and patronizing (appearing condescending and better than the patient). However, patients with mental illness are not somehow inferior to others; they do not necessarily have lower cognitive functioning; they are not less competent than others, nor out of control all the time. When the nurse believes any of these misconceptions, the resulting attitudes and behaviors can emerge in a microaggressive manner, erecting a wall between nurse and patient.

NURSING STRATEGIES FOR WORKING WITH THE MENTALLY ILL PATIENT

- *Clear and nonjudgmental conversation:* Use short sentences with clear meanings. Check yourself for biases, and make a conscious effort to see the patient as an individual needing your help.
- *Physical distance:* Maintain a physical distance from the patient that you are comfortable with, that is safe in the event of an unprovoked aggressive movement, and that also provides the patient with respect for his or her personal space.
- *Limit and boundary setting:* Be clear in your instructions when explaining what your expectations are, what you need from the patient, and what you can deliver to the patient.

- *Refocus or redirect attention:* If the patient begins to focus on an issue of fear, or an issue that is not pertinent to his or her care, gently refocus the patient's attention to the task at hand. For example, if you are interviewing a patient who suddenly starts talking about his mother's cancer diagnosis, acknowledge his concern and add a directive such as, "I hear how concerned you are about your mom's health; however, right now I need you to help me answer some of these questions about *your* health."

- *Honest, simple explanations of treatment options:* Patients may have had previous negative or positive experiences with treatments in environments similar to yours. These past experiences, both personal and those of others who have shared them with the patient, may provoke the patient to ask myriad questions about present and future care interventions. Listening to the questions and evaluating the nonverbal communications is the first necessity for the nurse; providing honest, simple explanations is the second. If you are unfamiliar with treatment modalities that the patient mentions, listen and let the patient know that you are unfamiliar with those specific interventions but you will get answers to any questions from someone who can provide more information.

- *Respect:* It is amazing how important and how impactful the demonstration of respect is to the patient with a psychiatric diagnosis. Treat your patient the way you would like to be treated, or the way you would like someone else to treat a member of your family.

- *Evidence-based management of presenting symptoms:* Find out what the patient is experiencing by asking about his or her symptoms. Find out what the patient thinks is causing the symptoms. Quite often the patient is very experienced at mitigating negative symptoms, or at least knows how others have helped to refocus on recovery. In this way, ask the questions that will allow you to learn from the patient about what has worked in the past, then collaborate with the patient to develop the care plan that will help the patient achieve his or her desired outcome.

- *Referral:* Know the mental health professionals who are available to you. Have a list of external references and referrals for the patient, from self-help organizations to professional mental health interventionists. Be aware of the multiple specialties (psychiatric nurse practitioners, social workers, physicians, mental health workers, counselors, etc.) who have continued their education to work specifically with this population.

- *Teamwork and education:* Become part of a team of health care providers who engage in increasing their knowledge of how to best care for our most vulnerable population—those with mental illness.

TAKE-AWAY

One in four Americans has a psychiatric disorder. Their disorders are brain-based illnesses over which they do not have control. More often than not these are your most vulnerable patients— people who count on health care providers to help them get their disease under control, and to assist them through recovery. Regardless of the specialized environment in which you have chosen to work, from obstetrics and women's health to geriatrics and hospice care, you *will* be taking care of patients who have psychiatric disorders. Learning the most you can about these disorders, and knowing when and whom to call for assistance, is essential to providing safe, evidence-based care.

Those of us working in the psychiatric field often say that the hardest thing for our patients to do is to ask for help, and the second hardest thing is to accept it. That may be true for members of the nursing profession, too. Knowing our strengths is important; knowing where we need to turn for help and when to rely on others is equally important. We are always stronger and better providers when we collaborate as a team, within nursing specialties, between nursing specialties, and among our diverse colleagues in health care practice.

Further Reading

American College of Emergency Physicians. (2014). Care of the psychiatric patient in the emergency department: A review of the literature. Retrieved from https://www.acep.org/uploadedFiles/ACEP/Clinical_and_Practice_Management/Resources/Mental_Health_and_Substance_Abuse/Psychiatric%20Patient%20Care%20in%20the%20ED%202014.pdf

American Psychiatric Association. (2013). *Diagnostic and statistical manual of mental disorders* (5th ed.). Arlington, VA: American Psychiatric Publishing.

American Psychiatric Association. (n.d.). Online assessment measures. Retrieved from https://www.psychiatry.org/psychiatrists/practice/dsm/dsm-5/online-assessment-measures

Boyd, M. A. (2015). *Psychiatric nursing contemporary practice* (5th ed.). Philadelphia, PA: Wolters Kluwer.

Boylan, C., & Waite, R. (2013). Psychiatric comorbidities in med/surg. *Advance Health for Nurses*. Retrieved from http://nursing.advanceweb.com

Bronheim, H. E., Fulop, G., Kunkel, E. J., Muskin, P. R., Schindler, B. A., Yates, W. R., . . . Stoudemire, A. (1998, August). Practice guidelines for psychiatric consultation in the general medical setting. *Academy of Psychosomatic Medicine, 39*, S8–S30.

Frost, M. (2006). The medical care of psychiatric inpatients: Suggestions for improvement. *The Internet Journal of Healthcare Administration, 4*(2). Retrieved from https://print.ispub.com/api/0/ispub-article/9240.

Halter, M. J., & Varcarolis, E. M. (2014). *Varcarolis' foundations of psychiatric mental health nursing: A clinical approach.* St. Louis, MO: Elsevier.

Levenson, J. L. (2007). Psychiatric issues in surgical patients part 1: General issues. *Primary Psychiatry, 14*(5), 35–39.

Naussbaum, A. (2013). *The pocket guide to the DSM-5 diagnostic exam.* Arlington, VA: American Psychiatric Publishing.

Perese, E. (2012). *Psychiatric advanced practice nursing: A biopsychosocial foundation for practice.* Philadelphia, PA: F. A. Davis.

Siegel, V. (2014). Outside the bedside comfort zone: Caring for a patient with psychiatric illness on a med/surg unit poses a unique set of challenges for nurses. Advance for NPs & PAs. Retrieved from http://nurse-practitioners-and-physician-assistants.advanceweb.com

Westerhof, G. J., & Keyes, C. L. M. (2010). Mental illness and mental health: The two continua model across the lifespan. *Journal of Adult Development, 17*(2), 110–119. doi:10.1007/s10804-009-9082-y

World Health Organization. (2003). Caring for children and adolescents with mental disorders: Setting WHO directions. Retrieved from http://www.who.int/mental_health/media/en/785.pdf.

Index

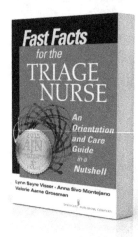
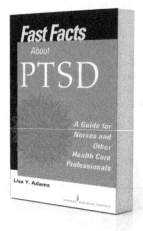
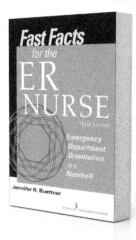
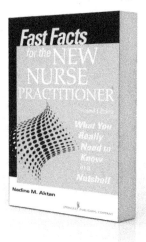